Field Guide to MEDLINE

Making Searching Simple

Field Guide to MEDLINE

Making Searching Simple

Christopher D. Stave, M.L.S.

Online and Instructional Services Coordinator
Lane Medical Library
Stanford University Medical Center
Stanford, California

 LIPPINCOTT WILLIAMS & WILKINS
A **Wolters Kluwer** Company
Philadelphia · Baltimore · New York · London
Buenos Aires · Hong Kong · Sydney · Tokyo

Acquisitions Editor: Richard Winters
Developmental Editors: Brian Brown and Michael Standen
Production Editor: Christiana Sahl
Manufacturing Manager: Tim Reynolds
Cover Designer: Jeane Norton
Compositor: Maryland Composition
Printer: Asia Pacific

© 2003 by LIPPINCOTT WILLIAMS & WILKINS
530 Walnut Street
Philadelphia, PA 19106 USA
LWW.com

Printed in China

Library of Congress Cataloging-in-Publication Data
Stave, Christopher D.
  Field guide to medline : making searching simple / Christopher D. Stave.
     p. cm. – (The field guide series)
  Includes bibliographical references and index
  ISBN 0-7817-3477-0
  1. MEDLINE. 2. Computer network resources. 3. Database searching. 4. Information retrieval–Study and teaching. I. Title. II. Field guide (Philadelphia, Pa.)
R858. S735 2003
025.06'61–dc21   2002066080

Publisher's Note: The Publisher wishes to thank the staff at Ovid Technologies, Inc., for their assistance in review of the final text and illustrations.

Care has been taken to confirm the accuracy of the information presented and to describe generally accepted practices. However, the author and publisher are not responsible for errors or omissions or for any consequences from application of the information–in this book and make no warranty, expressed or implied, with respect to the currency, completeness, or accuracy of the contents of the publication. Application of this information in a particular situation remains the professional responsibility of the practitioner.

The author and publisher have exerted every effort to ensure that drug selection and dosage set forth in this text are in accordance with current recommendations and practice at the time of publication. However, in view of ongoing research, changes in government regulations, and the constant flow of information relating to drug therapy and drug reactions, the reader is urged to check the package insert for each drug for any change in indications and dosage and for added warnings and precautions. This is particularly important when the recommended agent is a new or infrequently employed drug.

Some drugs and medical devices presented in this publication have Food and Drug Administration (FDA) clearance for limited use in restricted research settings. It is the responsibility of the health care provider to ascertain the FDA status of each drug or device planned for use in their clinical practice.

10 9 8 7 6 5 4 3 2 1

Contents

Preface

Acknowledgments

Preface

The *Field Guide to MEDLINE: Making Searching Simple* is designed for the busy health care professional who is looking for a practical, easy-to-use guide to MEDLINE via PubMed or Ovid. The bulk of the guide consists of MEDLINE search examples, which are illustrated by screen shots that are buttressed by simple, step-by-step instructions.

After ten years as a medical librarian, first at the Biomedical Library at the University of California, San Diego and then at the Lane Medical Library at the Stanford University Medical Center, I still marvel at the richness and complexity of MEDLINE. Despite the appearance of powerful new search tools and algorithms, effective MEDLINE searching continues to require knowledge, patience, and creativity. To say that I am still learning new things about MEDLINE searching may seem cliché, but it nevertheless is true. After all, the 11 million citations that comprise MEDLINE contain an amazing, and often intimidating, assortment of search tools—subject headings, subheadings, publication types, age groups, subsets, and so on. Their possible combinations are virtually limitless.

This is why MEDLINE searching is often an iterative process; in other words, when one strategy proves unproductive or simply fails outright, the user must be able to move smoothly and confidently to another. Hopefully, this guide will provide searchers with the flexibility to make these transitions easily and will enable them to adapt more effectively to the special and changing circumstances presented by each MEDLINE search.

At one time, MEDLINE was virtually the only substantive medical information resource available online. Needless to say, those days are long gone. Therefore, in order to avoid any sort of MEDLINE tunnel vision, the first chapter of the guide will provide a brief overview of the confusing, complicated, and rapidly-evolving universe of both free and fee-based online medical resources.

The second chapter provides both a description of the scope, content, and indexing of MEDLINE, and a review of some of the tools and strategies that are used to search it. The final two chapters apply these tools and strategies first to PubMed and then to Ovid MEDLINE. Specific information on printing, downloading, and e-mailing citations is also included.

The guide covers many, but not all, aspects of PubMed and Ovid MEDLINE. Moreover, the dynamic nature of web-based information resources means that the functionality and appearance of either system can change without warning (e.g., one day an icon in PubMed is labeled "Add to Clipboard" and the next, "Clip Add").

But why a *print* guide? Although the format may seem old-fashioned, I think well-designed, compact print guides are easier to use than most online help screens and many online tutorials. Help screens often compete for display space with the resource the user is searching, often forcing him or her to switch back and forth between windows. Stand-alone instructional tutorials, even though they are often informative and attractive, do not work particularly well as reference tools. In contrast, print guides do not obstruct computer monitors, and they can be marked up with a highlighter, placed in a lab coat pocket, or read over lunch in the cafeteria.

Thus, the *Field Guide to MEDLINE: Making Searching Simple* can be used as both a reference tool and a stand-alone instructional guide. In either case, I hope this text is practical, succinct, informative, and easy to use.

Christopher D. Stave

Acknowledgments

The notion of a practical, portable, attractively produced MEDLINE search guide grew from a series of discussions I had with Richard Winters, an Executive Editor at Lippincott Williams & Wilkins. We both felt that a well-designed and compact field guide could provide searchers with an easy-to-use resource whose content went beyond the standard cheat sheets or quick guides available at many medical libraries. Ultimately, Richard's interest and support convinced me to try to create just such a guide.

Describing the workings of web-based bibliographic databases would be difficult without a liberal dose of screen shots. Integrating these images with the blocks of text has been a challenging task, which was made immeasurably easier by the unstinting support and guidance of Christiana Sahl, the production editor for this book at Lippincott Williams & Wilkins. Additionally, Christiana provided ongoing editorial input that was both sorely needed and much appreciated.

My thanks are also extended to Timothy Roberts, Product Manger at Ovid Technologies, for his help in fine-tuning the chapter on Ovid MEDLINE.

I am particularly indebted to several members of the Bibliographic Services staff at the National Library of Medicine for their remarkably thorough critique of the chapter on PubMed. Their attention to detail was most impressive.

Finally, I would like to thank my friends and colleagues, including Marilyn Tinsley and Heidi Heilemann at Lane Medical Library and Brian Warling at the University of California, San Francisco, for their perceptive comments and helpful insights.

CHAPTER 1

Online Medical Information

What makes a search using MEDLINE[1] effective? What enables some searchers to devise dazzling strategies that conjure up wonderful results while others struggle with the most basic search operations or fret over large sets of irrelevant results (or none at all)?

Effective MEDLINE searchers are usually those with (a) a basic understanding of the breadth of the online medical information universe (e.g., what type of online information resources are available and which one is best suited to answer a particular question); (b) a firm grasp of the fundamental online search tools and strategies; (c) a clear sense of the structure and content of MEDLINE; and (d) proficiency with a particular MEDLINE system's attributes, features, and search modes. Search experience obviously helps, yet many MEDLINE searchers use crude or ineffective tactics for years because they are unaware of more efficient and more productive approaches.

This chapter provides a brief review of the universe of online information resources, of which MEDLINE is just one part.

OVERVIEW

The growth of the World Wide Web has had an enormous and well-documented impact on how information is accessed and disseminated, and nowhere is this truer than in health and medicine (1). Textbooks and journals that once were accessible primarily in print or, alternatively, on CD-ROM are now increasingly available via the Web. Powerful new drug information resources, many of which contain the entire contents of stand-alone drug texts (e.g., *Physicians' Desk Reference, MARTINDALE: The Complete Drug Reference*) are offered on the Web, usually for a fee. Clinical practice guidelines can be found in online depositories (e.g., the National Guideline Clearinghouse) or within a sponsoring organization's website (e.g., American Academy of Pediatrics). Web-based "prefiltered" evidence-based medicine databases that analyze and synthesize the medical literature are growing rapidly in popularity. Not surprisingly, several commercial ventures have collected many of these dispersed, heterogeneous resources into self-contained systems with global search capabilities.

Following is a brief overview of these and other resources, along with occasional comments about their relative advantages and disadvantages. Please remember that the labels *databases, electronic journals* (e-journals), and so on are to some extent approximations of rapidly evolving, frequently overlapping types of resources. In other words, Web-based resources often share similar characteristics, thus precluding precise segregation; for example, some e-journal websites are beginning to resemble Web "portals" because they include links to medical databases, online continuing education courses, employment information, alerting services, and other similar information.

---

[1]MEDLINE, PubMed, MeSH, Loansome Doc, AIDSLINE, and BIOETHICS-LINE are registered trademarks to the United States National Library of Medicine.

Databases

What is a *database*? The types of databases described in this field guide are primarily bibliographic, and they may be thought of as *files* containing *records* (e.g., journal article citations) that represent a *document* or other work (e.g., a journal article, book, or book chapter). The database records in turn are comprised of *fields* that contain information about the document (e.g., author, title, journal). Data from these fields generally are placed into searchable indices (e.g., author index, title index).

Database *publishers* create databases. These publishers (both profit and nonprofit) are primarily, although not exclusively, responsible for (a) determining a database's thematic scope, (b) selecting what types of documents are indexed (e.g., journal articles, books, book chapters, or meeting abstracts), (c) establishing quality criteria for inclusion (i.e., MEDLINE indexes some journals but not others), (d) creating indexing policies, (e) developing a thesaurus of subjects (although not all databases have subject headings or a thesaurus), and (f) leasing or distributing electronic copies or printed indices of the database.

Commercial database *vendors* license the content of databases such as MEDLINE. These vendors, including Ovid, provide a search interface for the database, and they may include value-added features, such as links to full-text journal articles.

Other types of databases, such as the government's statistical databases, are primarily numeric. Some, such as the *Cochrane Database of Systematic Reviews*, provide full text.

Bibliographic Databases

MEDLINE, BIOSIS Previews, EMBASE, and PsycINFO are typical examples of bibliographic databases. Most contain citations representing printed works (e.g., journal articles, books, book chapters, and reports) in a particular discipline or group of disciplines. The publishers of these databases generally adhere to a definite and sometimes quite rigorous screening process for the materials they index.

The size of these databases has given rise to a number of different search tools and aids. Among the most important are the extensive subject vocabularies (sometimes called "controlled" vocabularies) that database publishers may create to help searchers improve the efficiency and accuracy of their searches. The vocabularies are published in online or print "thesauri." They are either unique to a particular database, or they may be shared among several different databases (e.g., MEDLINE's Medical Subject Headings [MeSH] are used to index MEDLINE *and* CANCERLIT).

These databases are often the resources of choice for searches where exhaustive coverage of the topic is critical (e.g., metaanalyses). In addition, when searches of more specialized databases (e.g., the evidence-based medicine collections) fail to produce any relevant information or if the information contained within them seems questionable, switching to some of the aforementioned bibliographic databases may be appropriate. Keep in mind, however, that no single database indexes everything.

Citation Databases

Citation databases, such as the Science Citation Index, are an interesting variation on the usual bibliographic database structure. They can be used as a standard bibliographic database or as a "citation" database that is designed to reveal "who is citing whom." For example, one can enter basic information about a particular journal article (e.g., author, journal, year, page number), and the citation database will list how many times that article has been cited and by whom.

Because ISI is the only company to produce this type of information, subscription costs can be rather high. However, for faculty who are seeking tenure and who therefore wish to quantify the impact of their work on their respective disciplines, a citation report can prove invaluable. Citation databases can also provide a useful adjunct to standard database searching. For example, if a search of MEDLINE pulls up only one or two relevant records, these records can then be plugged into a citation database to discover who is citing them. The expectation of the searcher is that the content of the *citing* articles might reflect the content of the original *cited* article. Most large universities have subscriptions to at least the print versions of these indexes, and many are beginning to subscribe to the Web-based versions as well.

Prefiltered or Synthesized Bibliographic Databases

The astonishing numbers of records added to the primary literature databases make efficient separation of the "best" information from the rest difficult for health care professionals. This is one reason for the growth of "prefiltered" or "synthesized" bibliographic databases.

Evidence-based medicine databases, including the *Cochrane Database of Systematic Reviews*, the *Database of Abstracts of Reviews of Effectiveness*, the *American College of Physicians (ACP) Journal Club*, and *Clinical Evidence* (from the BMJ Publishing Group), evaluate and synthesize studies that report on the effectiveness of a treatment or prevention strategy. In theory, these collections can be used to retrieve the "best" information without running exhaustive searches in the standard bibliographic databases.

Practice guideline collections are yet another vehicle for the distribution of synthesized clinical research. Because such a vast number of associations, societies, and government organizations distribute these publications, locating a specific guideline is often difficult. Fortunately, the Agency for Healthcare Research and Quality, in partnership with the American Medical Association and the American Association of Health Plans, created the National Guideline Clearinghouse to facilitate access to clinical practice guidelines. Each guideline record includes summaries and syntheses of the guideline, as well as information on the availability of the full text. The Clearinghouse is searchable on the Web at no charge (http://www.guideline.gov/).

Many collections, however, are still relatively small, and searches often retrieve few or no results. On the other hand, the small size of the databases makes searching relatively easy.

When to Use These Databases

The synthesized databases, such as the Cochrane Database of Systematic Reviews, are often excellent starting points (if one has access to them) when searching for information on the effectiveness of *intervention X* on *disease or condition Y* (e.g., *acupuncture AND asthma*). If these databases fail to answer the question or if the information that is retrieved appears questionable, then the user might need to switch to one of the standard bibliographic databases, such as MEDLINE.

Online Catalogs

Online catalogs, which are the successor to card catalogs, are repositories of records representing the monographic, journal, audio, audiovisual, and software (sometimes) collection of a particular organization.

When to Use Online Catalogs

These catalogs can be used to locate books, journals, audiovisuals, and other materials. Although one may be able to access the online catalog of a nearby medical library via the Web, he or she may not have borrowing privileges. The user should check with the library first. If unsure of which medical library is nearest, this information can be found by visiting the Web-based National Network of Libraries of Medicine (NLM) "library finder" at http://nnlm.gov/members/.

If the item is not found at a local medical library, the user may try the NLM online catalog LOCATORplus at http://locatorplus.gov/. He or she should remember that requests for materials from the NLM's collection must be processed through a library. For more information about borrowing from the NLM, the reader should contact the nearest public or medical library.

If one is looking to purchase the item, it can be ordered through an online "store," such as Amazon (http://www.amazon.com/) or purchased through a university bookstore with a medical textbook collection.

Electronic Journals

Electronic medical journals are usually (although not always) the online equivalent of a print journal. The following advantages are obvious: e-journals are accessible via the Web; they often appear before their print counterparts; they cannot be shelved in the wrong place; they do not have articles torn out; they do not have to be sent to the bindery; and they cannot be "checked out," although user licenses often do restrict access to a finite number of simultaneous users. Also, many e-journals contain information unavailable in their print counterparts, such as links to preprints, membership directories, employment information, continuing medical education (CME), and much more.

Not surprisingly, the explosive growth in the number of e-journals has had a dramatic impact on the accessibility and distribution of medical information. Stanford University's Lane Medical Library, for example, has acquired e-journal subscriptions to more than two-thirds of its collection to the great satisfaction of its patrons. Most of these journals are supplied by publishers (e.g., Elsevier and Academic Press) and resource aggregators (e.g., Ovid and MD Consult) or via online "presses" (e.g., HighWire Press). Some journals are free, but most are not. Adding to the complexity, single journals may be supplied by multiple sources; for example, *The Lancet* can be accessed from ScienceDirect (Elsevier) and Journals@Ovid (Ovid Technologies), as well as directly from the Lancet Publishing Group. Depending on the system, the appearance of the journal articles may vary. Access restrictions also vary. Some require user names and passwords, some are restricted to a particular site or institution, and some utilize all of these. Both users (and librarians) may have difficulty in keeping track of the resulting user names, log-in identifications, and passwords.

Sometimes simply determining whether a journal is available online can offer a significant challenge. Although features like PubMed's LinkOut and Ovid's OpenLinks have expanded the number of links between database citations and electronic full-text articles dramatically, access often involves a subscription or fee. When a user is in doubt about the availability of a journal, he or she should check the institution's online catalog (if affiliated with an institution), contact a nearby medical library, or use a search engine (e.g., Google at http://www.google.com/) to visit the journal's website.

Other issues will continue to challenge and vex e-journal subscribers for the foreseeable future; for example, how will archives of electronic journals be accessed when subscriptions are canceled? How do institutions establish pricing structures relative to individual subscribers? How is access (on-site versus off-site) to a journal managed and priced? These issues notwithstanding, the benefits of e-journals are immense.

When to Use E-Journals
In addition to providing the full text of journal articles, e-journals often contain substantial value-added information. Journals, such as the *British Medical Journal*, provide instructions for authors, alerting services, access to MEDLINE, information about upcoming meetings and conferences, and career planning advice, among others. Clearly, e-journals have the potential to offer far more than their print counterparts.

Electronic Books

Web-accessible textbooks are generally available in a stand-alone (e.g., Harrison's Online) or bundled format (e.g., part of a medical information collection, such as those available through Books@Ovid, MD Consult, eMedicine, Skolar, and MD). PubMed's *Bookshelf* provides a searchable set of several biomedical textbooks that link key phrases to citations within PubMed.).

Probably the greatest problem with electronic books (e-books) is devising effective searching strategies. Strategies that work for standard bibliographic databases may not necessarily work for books. Different e-book publishers have grappled with this problem in different ways; some allow searches only of the tables of contents and book indices, whereas others actually provide searching of the text itself.

Precise definitions of what actually constitutes an electronic textbook fail when they are applied to resources like UpToDate and WebMD Scientific American Medicine. UpToDate describes itself as a clinical "reference tool" containing topic reviews written by experts. The reviews address specific clinical issues and provide detailed recommendations. The Web version of WebMD Scientific American Medicine (SAM) is the electronic manifestation of a loose-leaf general medicine reference resource. SAM is updated monthly.

When to Use e-Books
When an integrated summary of research on a particular subject is needed, e-books are a good source. As currency can be an issue, supplemental searches of an online bibliographic database may be indicated.

Drug Information

The Web provides access to an astonishing amount of information about drugs. Some of the information is free, while some require a subscription or fee. The quality of drug information on the Web is variable.

Some of the larger fee-based resources include Lexi-Comp, MicroMedex, and Clinical Pharmacology 2000 (the last of these currently is free to physicians). Lexi-Comp's Clinical Reference Library contains a variety of drug handbooks. MicroMedex includes a rich collection of drug databases. Some resources, such as Lexi-Drugs and ePocrates Rx, are designed for Palm OS-compatible handheld computers; these cover commonly prescribed medications.

A popular source of free information about drugs that is geared toward either the patient or consumer is that of the United States Pharmacopoeia Drug Information (USP DI), which has an "Advice for the Patient" resource that is available through MEDLINEplus, a consumer health information Web portal.

When to Use Drug Information Resources on the Web
If one is looking for information about a particular drug—dosage, interactions, pharmacokinetics, side effects, or other information—these resources can help.

News and Current Awareness

Medical information aggregators constantly strive to find new ways of providing busy health care professionals with current news and information quickly and efficiently. Some systems provide the text of the news portions of popular medical journals, medically relevant news from Reuters, or summaries of medical articles from popular newspapers and magazines.

Another approach for remaining current involves storing database search strategies. For example, searchers can use Ovid's AutoAlert to save their MEDLINE search strategies. These strategies are regularly and automatically run against newly added citations. Any "hits" are sent to the searcher's e-mail address. PubMed offers a similar service, except that the user must rerun the stored search (see "Storing Searches Using the Cubby" in Chapter 3).

When to Use Stored Searches
If you have an ongoing interest in a particular medical topic, the search storage features in Ovid and PubMed are invaluable.

Continuing Medical Education

Like electronic textbooks, CME is often supplied as part of a larger, bundled information system. In most cases, users register with the service, take the course, perhaps take a test, and submit the answers; they then are rewarded with a certificate of some sort, usually for a fee. Interactive case-based approaches, like those provided by MedCases, are particularly popular.

When to Use Continuing Medical Education
Use CME to review basic skills, to learn new skills, and to fulfill licensure requirements.

Decision Support Systems

As the name implies, decision support systems (DSSs) are used to facilitate and supplement clinical (and sometimes nonclinical) decision making. Although most of the online resources listed in this chapter could be construed as "decision support," DSSs are usually more directly or more explicitly integrated into the decision-making process. Some of these systems link with the electronic patient record or order entry system to provide health care providers with a variety of suggestions, alerts, and reminders. One of the most popular applications of DSS is its use as a drug prescription safeguard that is designed to spot "red flags," such as potentially dangerous drug combinations or drug dosages that exceed certain parameters (2).

Variations on these systems include stand-alone DSS tools, such as Med-Weaver, DXplain, Iliad, and QMR. DXplain, for example, is described by its website as " . . . a decision support system that uses a set of clinical findings (signs, symptoms, laboratory data) to produce a ranked list of diagnoses, which might explain (or be associated with) the clinical manifestations" (3). The system is interactive, and it regularly updates its list of diagnoses as new data are entered by the user.

When to Use Decision Support Systems
The uses vary widely. Diagnostic decision support resources like DXplain are particularly popular as clinical education tools.

Medical Association, Society, and Government Websites

The websites of reputable medical associations, societies, and organizations can be invaluable sources of high-quality information. These sites often include position statements, practice guidelines, consumer health information, online journals, meeting and conference information, and CME modules. Generally, the easiest way to locate the website of one of these is via a search engine such as Google (simply type in the name of the organization and click Go).

Government websites provide an enormous amount of health-related information, much of which is available at no charge. Databases of clinical trials, compendia of grant information, mountains of statistical information, and United States Food and Drug Administration (FDA) approval reports on drugs and devices are all available on the web. The trick is getting to the specific piece of data that is needed. One problem is the awkwardness and imprecision of the local search engines of some government websites. If one cannot find what he or she is looking for on the site itself, another strategy is to try a search engine like Google, using the advanced search interface to target Web pages within a specific domain (e.g., fda.gov).

When to Use Medical Association, Society, and Government Websites
Society and association sites are often excellent sources of information about upcoming meetings, abstracts of past meetings, membership directories, news of relevance to the membership, publications, and position statements.

For practice guidelines and consumer health information in particular, pre-sorted clearinghouses and consumer health collections (e.g., National Guideline Clearinghouse and MEDLINEplus) are some of the best places to start.

Not surprisingly, government sites are rich sources of statistical information. For medicine and health statistics, the websites for the Centers for Disease Control and Prevention (CDC) and the National Center for Health Statistics (NCHS is part of the CDC) are particularly useful. As has already been mentioned, locating the right information can be quite a challenge. *Contact a medical librarian if initial efforts prove unproductive.*

Consumer Health Information

Vast quantities of "consumer health" information have flooded the Web in recent years. Predictably, the quality is variable. Various associations, societies, universities, and government organizations have created their own consumer health clearinghouses in an attempt to separate the accurate and trustworthy information from the rest. A notable effort is the NLM's MEDLINEplus, a collection of publications, dictionaries, encyclopedias, directories, news, drug databases, and more. Commercial medical Web portals (or *vortals*) often offer large collections of consumer-oriented and patient-oriented handouts and pamphlets. (See "Portals and Vortals" below.)

Disease-specific electronic discussion groups can provide patients with helpful information, but they also can be sources of erroneous or misleading information, particularly when untested and unproved treatments are recommended.

When to Use Consumer Health Information

Consumer health information sites can be great sources of background information on diseases and medications, but their quality can vary greatly—use with caution.

Services and Applications

A vital part of some commercial medical websites is the collection of services they offer to the health care professional. These services can be quite elaborate, and they may include systems for equipment purchase, electronic medical record management, billing, and insurance eligibility checking. Other services, such as research assistance and document delivery, may be available to the physician or health care professional from a medical library for free or at a reduced rate. Some medical websites also include links to electronic tools and applications, including calculators, nomograms, educational aids, and drug downloads for personal digital assistants (PDAs).

Document Delivery

To find the perfect MEDLINE record is one thing; to obtain the article is another. Various document delivery options are available to the physician, the most notable of which is the Loansome Doc service via PubMed. Physicians must register with a local medical library and pay a small fee to obtain articles through Loansome Doc.

Usually, affiliation with a hospital or medical center qualifies the requester for some kind of document delivery (possibly for a fee). However, for the general public, the situation is less clear. Recently, links to several commercial document delivery providers were added to PubMed. Not surprisingly, fees, registration requirements, and delivery methods for these services vary. One may contact the local medical library to find out more about document delivery.

Calculators and Nomograms

Growing numbers of health-oriented calculators, nomograms, regimens, scores, tables, and algorithms are appearing across the Web. Sites like eMedicine and ePocrates provide access, often for free, to many of these tools.

Personal Digital Assistant Downloads

The popularity of handheld computers, or PDAs, has greatly intrigued electronic medical information suppliers. Downloads of drug information, calculators and nomograms, electronic textbooks, journal tables of contents, flash cards, and even full-motion videos are widely available, either free or for a fee. One of the more popular downloads for PDAs is the ePocrates drug database, ePocrates Rx (see preceding section, "Drug Information").

Portals and Vortals

The past several years have witnessed an explosion in the number of medically oriented websites that integrate a diverse array of resources into a single online environment. These sites can provide access to virtually every resource described in this chapter—online medical books, e-journals, drug information, news, CME, and DSS. The richness of the sites varies, but the strategy is the same—to satisfy all (or almost all) of a busy health professional's medical information needs. For fee-based services, in particular, the idea seems to be to keep the subscriber corralled within the confines of the website by offering enough services and features so that he or she has little need to go elsewhere. These sites are distinguished from general collections of resources like Yahoo! (often called *horizontal portals*) by the somewhat unpleasant term *vortals*. Vortals, or *vertical portals*, focus on a specific discipline or specialty.

Some of these vortals are fee based, requiring a subscription to gain access to *any* of the resources. One of the big selling points of these sites is the ability to run global searches across the entire collection. In other words, a single search statement can be run simultaneously against textbooks, journals, patient education pamphlets, and other resources. This kind of searching is by definition inexact—searching a textbook can require different strategies from those needed for searching a medical database like MEDLINE. Instead, global searching is a way to get a quick sense of where most of the information might reside. If more precision is required, accessing the specific resource is better (e.g., a special "practice guideline" search interface provides options unavailable in the global search mode).

Characterizing vortals with great precision is difficult as hybrids abound. Some sites contain a mix of free and fee-based resources; WebMD is a typical example. Some sites are annotated and peer-reviewed collections of links to other medical resources, of which BioSites and Medical Matrix are two examples. Browsing through the different sites (many of the fee-based sites provide free trials) is probably the best way for an individual to discover which ones he or she prefers.

Search Engines

Web search engines are indispensable. The best can extract useful information from a mountain of irrelevant muck. Google, for example, with its simple search interface and dazzling relevancy-ranking algorithms, is, in the author's experience, particularly effective.

The features offered by search engines vary. Some provide supplemental collections of links organized by subject (similar to portals like Yahoo!); some allow the user to target specific types of media (e.g., pictures, movies, sound); and some allow the searcher to perform simultaneous searches across multiple search engines (e.g., MetaCrawler).

When to Use Search Engines

Search engines can often find information that one cannot find in "traditional" online sources. For locating a meeting abstract, a profile of a colleague, a picture of a cirrhotic liver, or even a list of plumbers in Des Moines, search engines often are the fastest, most efficient solution.

Not surprisingly, the quality of the information retrieved by search engines varies. For high-quality peer-reviewed articles, for example, standard bibliographic databases like MEDLINE perform better.

THE FUTURE

The growth of new medical information is fast outpacing the ability of clinicians (and consumers) to stay current. As a result, the number of predigested, preanalyzed online information collections appears to be growing.

One growing trend is toward simple search interfaces backed by extremely sophisticated search engines (e.g., Google, PubMed). Searchers using these engines often retrieve excellent information quickly and painlessly with less intervention or mediation on the part of information professionals.

Which online resources will survive is anyone's guess; however, the supposition that sites with well-designed search interfaces, affordable subscription rates, regular updates, and high-quality content are much more likely to succeed seems reasonable.

REFERENCES

1. Taylor H, Leitman R. New data show Internet, website and email usage by physicians all increasing. *HealthCare News* 2001;1:1–3.
2. Lippman H. Clinical decision support: beyond cookbook medicine. *Hippocrates* 2000;14:33–37.
3. DXPlain home page. Available at: http://dxplain.mgh.harvard.edu/. Accessed June 2002.

CHAPTER 2

MEDLINE: Overview of Content, Basic Tools, and Search Strategies

This chapter provides searchers with a brief overview of MEDLINE and a quick summary of some common online search tools and strategies. More specifically, this chapter will accomplish the following:
1. Review the history, structure, and indexing of MEDLINE;
2. Explain the function of several key online search tools;
3. Describe the elements of an effective search;
4. Describe six popular MEDLINE search strategies;
5. Summarize the relative advantages of PubMed and Ovid MEDLINE;
6. Provide useful search tips to consider *before* running a search.

MEDLINE

MEDLINE is probably the best known and most widely used biomedical database available today. Free to anyone with access to the Internet, MEDLINE is often considered by most clinicians, researchers, patients, and consumers, whether rightly or wrongly, the biomedical information resource of choice.

Content and Coverage

According to the National Library of Medicine (NLM)'s *MEDLINE Factsheet*, MEDLINE's subject coverage includes "Basic biomedical research and the clinical sciences since 1966 including nursing, dentistry, veterinary medicine, pharmacy, allied health, and pre-clinical sciences. MEDLINE also covers life sciences that are vital to practitioners, researchers, and educators, including some aspects of biology, environmental science, marine biology, plant and animal science as well as biophysics and chemistry. Increased coverage of life sciences began in 2000" (1).

MEDLINE's journal coverage is international, including some 4,000 journals from 70 countries. Most articles are in English, or they at least contain English abstracts written by the authors. MEDLINE currently contains more than 11 million records, to which 40,000 new records are added each month. OLDMEDLINE, available through LOCATORplus (see "LOCATORplus" in Appendix 2: Other Databases and Resources), roughly covers 1958 through 1965.

The NLM has changed its policy toward its online databases so that collections will be *format* based rather than *subject* based. In other words, journal article records from specialty databases, such as AIDSLINE and BIOETHICS-LINE, will be merged with MEDLINE. Nonjournal records from these databases (e.g., books, book chapters, and meeting abstracts) will be accessible from LOCATORplus or the NLM Gateway.

Although MEDLINE currently covers 1966 to the present, OLDMEDLINE, another database, goes a bit further back. Searchable through the NLM Gateway, OLDMEDLINE represents the 1960 through 1965 *Cumulated Index*

Medicus and the 1958 through 1959 *Current List of Medical Literature*. Records for this database do *not* include abstracts. (**NOTE:** MEDLINE contains about 100,000 records for articles *published* in 1965 that were not *indexed* until 1966.)

History

MEDLINE is the electronic successor to a venerable 120-year-old print-based index known as *Index Medicus*. Created in 1879, *Index Medicus* has gone through a number of changes over the course of its long history. One of the most important of these was the integration of the Index into an electronic management system called MEDLARS (Medical Literature, Analysis, and Retrieval System). MEDLINE, short for MEDLARS Online, is the searchable database portion of MEDLARS. MEDLINE grew to include two other indexes—the *Index to Dental Literature* and the *International Nursing Index*. The amazing accessibility of this database called into question the need for continued publication of the print indexes, and, in the summer of 2000, the NLM announced that it would cease publication of its annual cumulated index, the *Cumulated Index Medicus*.

Value-Added Content and Services

Most of the searching systems that provide access to MEDLINE offer a variety of supplemental resources and services (e.g., links to electronic journals, online textbooks, other databases, and document delivery services).

MEDLINE INDEXING

What makes MEDLINE arguably the best biohealth database for searching *anywhere* is the amazing amount of value-added indexing information packed into its 11 million records. These records contain not only the usual collection of bibliographic information, (e.g., author, title, journal) but also medical subject headings, subheadings, publication types, grant numbers, age groups, and much more. These extra bits of information provide a rich array of search points for those savvy enough to use them.

MEDLINE indexers are responsible for the creation of most of this information. Approximately 100 indexers perform subject analysis for MEDLINE. New indexers hold at least a bachelor's degree in the life sciences, and they are required to attend a 2-week-long course in NLM indexing principles. Quality control is enhanced by software programs designed to improve indexing consistency and accuracy. Indexers must understand the subject content of the articles they index, and they then must represent the substantive portions of this content with Medical Subject Headings (MeSH) (approximately 10 to 12 per article).

Medical Subject Headings

Like most other controlled vocabularies, MeSH are a standardized collection of terms that represent the substantive content of a particular work. More than 19,000 medical subject headings are available to indexers at the NLM. The breadth of coverage is impressive; the MeSH include diseases, drugs, diagnostic tests, various organisms, aspects of health care, and much more. All MeSH terms are organized hierarchically, and they fall under one or more broad subject headings (e.g., Diseases, Signs and Symptoms, and Anatomy). Indexers usually add 10 to 12 MeSH terms per record, and they then identify two or three of these terms as major themes within the article. The headings are updated annually; outdated MeSHs are discarded or renamed, and new MeSHs are added.

The MeSH terms are also designed for specificity. For example, an indexer would index an article about migraine with the MeSH term *migraine* rather than with the more general MeSH term *headache disorders*. Experienced searchers use this characteristic of MEDLINE to enhance the precision of their searches.

Finally, MeSH terms are intended to be standardized representations of a particular concept. For example, articles on kidney stones are indexed with the MeSH *kidney calculi*, regardless of variations in an author's terminology (e.g., *renal stones, renal calculi, nephrolithiasis*).

Advantages and Disadvantages

Advantage One
Often, MeSH will retrieve records that do not necessarily mention the search topic in the title or abstract. Because MEDLINE indexers actually scan the articles they index, an article may not have mentioned the search topic in the title or abstract; if the search topic is a key part of the article, however, the indexers will represent it with MeSH terms. This is particularly useful when retrieving records with "cute" but meaningless titles, especially when these records lack abstracts.

Advantage Two
As was mentioned above, MeSH terms are intended to represent a particular concept uniquely. Without MeSH, searchers would be compelled to search batches of synonymous terms (e.g., *renal stones, kidney stones, renal calculi, and nephrolithiasis*).

Advantage Three
The hierarchic arrangement of MeSH is a great advantage. If, for example, one is searching for articles that examine the effectiveness of cephalosporins on respiratory tract infections, he or she could locate and search the MeSH terms for each cephalosporin (e.g., cefaclor, cefadroxil, cefamandole, cefazolin, cefixime) and gather them into a set. This, however, would be a waste of time. Instead, searching the MeSH term *cephalosporins* retrieves the narrower headings, including *cefaclor, cefadroxil*, and others. A search of the MeSH heading Respiratory Tract Infections retrieves *bronchitis, pneumonia, pinusitis, influenza*, and *rhinitis*. Furthermore, if these headings have their own narrower headings (e.g., *sinusitis* includes *ethmoid sinusitis, frontal sinusitis, sphenoid sinusitis*, and *maxillary sinusitis*), these would be included in the search. Therefore, to run the search, the user can simply combine the MeSH terms as follows: *cephalosporins AND respiratory tract infections*.

This process, which is called *exploding*, is one of the most powerful tools available to the MEDLINE searcher. In many, but not all, MEDLINE search systems, exploding occurs automatically.

13

Disadvantage One

Indexing inconsistency can be a problem. Research has shown that different indexers use different combinations of MeSH terms to describe the content of the same article (2).

Disadvantage Two

Not all concepts are represented by MeSH. For new topics to acquire equivalent MeSH terms takes time. Until that happens, the user should employ free-text searching (include variant terminology).

Subheadings or Qualifiers

Experienced MEDLINE searchers often use MeSH subheadings as a way to represent more completely a particular aspect of a topic. Searchers can choose from more than 80 subheadings and can link them directly to a MeSH term. Some examples of some of the more popular subheadings include Adverse Effects, Complications, Drug Therapy, Economics, Epidemiology, Diagnosis, Etiology, Prevention and Control, Therapy, and Trends. Subheadings usually apply to particular types of MeSH; for example, a searcher cannot link Administration and Dosage directly to the MeSH term *anterior cruciate ligament*.

Publication Types

Another technique for increasing the precision of a search involves the use of publication types. For example, a search on *aminoglycosides AND urinary tract infections* could be limited to articles indexed as randomized controlled trials, review articles, or metaanalyses.

Check Tags

The term *check tags* is a holdover from the days when indexers literally "checked off" basic information about an article as it was indexed. These tags include Human, Animal, Male, Female, Case Report, Comparative Study, and so on. The Human check tag is particularly useful, and it can be used in a search to focus on human studies.

Subsets

Topic, journal, and citation status subsets provide another method for narrowing the scope of the search. For example, the Core Clinical Journals subset limits the search to 120 high-impact clinical journals, many of which are subscribed to by small-sized to medium-sized hospital libraries.

BASIC SEARCH TOOLS

The following basic search tools belong in every online searcher's toolkit: truncation, adjacency, Boolean operators, and nesting. Although they are obviously useful when searching MEDLINE, these handy tools often work with other online resources, from electronic textbooks to Web search engines. The system-specific applications vary somewhat (e.g., PubMed uses an asterisk [*] for truncation; Ovid uses a dollar sign [$]), but the principles are basically the same.

Boolean Operators

The Boolean operators *AND, OR, NOT* are the three little workhorses of online searching. These operators can be used to narrow, broaden, or exclude search terms.

AND	Both terms must occur
	amoxicillin AND pneumonia
OR	Either some or all of the terms can occur
	gourds OR pumpkins OR squashes
NOT	One term but not the other
	aids NOT hearing

In most systems, Boolean operators are processed from left to right. The order is important because a poorly designed search statement can retrieve unexpected, misleading, or incorrect results. The following example illustrates a common mistake:

aspirin AND heart attack OR myocardial infarction.

Aspirin AND heart attack is processed first and retrieves a hypothetical set of, say, 100 records. Next, *myocardial infarction* generates 30,000 records. The two sets are combined with *OR* for a set of 30,050 records. (This number is not 30,100 because 50 records in the first set were also in the second set, and duplicates are eliminated.) Clearly, these results would not be what the searcher expected. The following would be a better search:

heart attack OR myocardial infarction AND aspirin.

Heart attack OR myocardial infarction retrieves 30,450 records. *Aspirin* retrieves 7,100. Combining the two sets with *AND* retrieves 250 records, a much more reasonable and manageable result.

Nesting or Using Parentheses

Parentheses often alleviate the confusion that arises when using multiple Boolean operators. The use of parentheses, which is rather quaintly known as nesting, allows the user to control more precisely the order in which the elements of the search are processed. How? Most search systems process what occurs in parentheses *before* anything else. Therefore, the poorly designed search *aspirin AND heart attack OR myocardial infarction* could be improved either by changing the order of the search terms (see above) or through the strategic placement of parentheses as follows:

aspirin AND (heart attack OR myocardial infarction).

Heart attack OR myocardial infarction retrieves 30,450 records. *Aspirin* retrieves 7,100. Combining both with *AND,* as is shown above, retrieves 250 records. The "deepest" parentheses are processed first as in the following example:

aspirin AND (heart attack OR (MI OR myocardial infarction)).

NOTE: With complex searches, keeping track of parentheses is sometimes difficult. Checking to ensure that the number of left parentheses equals the number of right parentheses can help.

Truncation and Wild Cards

Truncation and, to a lesser extent, wild cards are popular and powerful online search tools. A truncation symbol allows the searcher to truncate a word, usually at any point following the first three characters. Thus, a search of *allerg** will retrieve records containing *allergy*, *allergens*, *allergic*, and so on.

Some systems, such as Ovid, provide a set of characters called *wild cards*. These symbols usually replace one, two, or no characters. For example, *wom#n* retrieves both *women* and *woman*. *Colo#r* retrieves both *color* and *colour*. As this handbook describes later, Ovid provides significantly more truncation and wild card options than PubMed.

Adjacency and Proximity

The ability to specify nearness or distance between search terms is provided by adjacency or proximity operators. Phrase searching is perhaps the most common example of adjacency, which is one word next to another (e.g., *mad cow disease*). Ovid does a good job of phrase searching.

Ovid also enables the use of proximity operators to locate one search term within *X* number of words of another search term in any order. For example, one could locate the term *costs* within five words (in any order) of the phrase *cardiac rehabilitation*.

Relevancy Ranking

Search results can be listed in order of most relevant in several ways. The most obvious and most common is reverse chronological; that is, the most recent records are listed first. PubMed also has a remarkable feature called "Related Article" that retrieves a precalculated set of citations that are similar to or "related" to a selected citation. The related records are listed in the order of the most relevant first. The algorithm that determines relevancy considers a number of factors, including term frequency and term position within the record (e.g., if the terms appear in the title, the record is probably more relevant than one in which the terms appear in the abstract).

Distantly related to this algorithm is Ovid's "frequency" feature, which allows a searcher to retrieve records based solely on term frequency. The underlying principle is quite intuitive: the more a search term appears in a record, the greater is the chance that the record is relevant to the search.

ELEMENTS OF AN EFFECTIVE SEARCH

The most effective MEDLINE searchers know how to formulate their searches in ways that take full advantage of MEDLINE's tools and features. They understand the implications of different strategies on retrieval and how to reformulate these strategies quickly when necessary. They also know when to use free-text searching, when to use MeSH, and when to use both in combination. The following section highlights some of the elements that searchers manipulate when developing a search strategy, and it describes a popular method for calculating a search strategy's relative effectiveness.

Free-Text Searches

Free-text searches, often called *keyword* searches, usually involve searches of words or phrases in multiple fields (e.g., title, abstract). The main problem with most free-text searching is imprecision. For example, simply because the phrase *cervical spine fractures* occurs in an abstract, this does not mean that *cervical spine fractures* is a significant theme of the article (e.g., an article stating that future studies on external fixation should focus on cervical spine fractures). In addition, free-text searching means that one may need to include variant terminology for a topic to increase retrieval (e.g., *stone OR calculi*).

On the other hand, a well-constructed free-text search can retrieve records that a subject search misses. For example, in PubMed, a free-text search can retrieve *in process* and *supplied by publisher* records that lack *any* MeSH terms. In addition, a free-text search sometimes retrieves citations that have been inconsistently indexed by MEDLINE indexers.

Subject Headings

Although the advantages of MeSH were described earlier, looking at how subject headings relate to the other elements of a search can be useful. For example, if one is searching for *adult respiratory distress syndrome*, he or she could run a search of MEDLINE using the heading Respiratory Distress Syndrome, Adult. If this search retrieves 7,000 records, the user can be reasonably sure that Respiratory Distress Syndrome, Adult is a topic (either a central topic or one that is more peripheral) of each of the 7,000 articles. If this were not the case, the indexers would not have bothered indexing the records with Respiratory Distress Syndrome, Adult. The search can be represented as follows:

respiratory distress syndrome, adult [mesh]

What happens next depends on how much time the user has, how much he or she knows about MEDLINE, how much he or she knows about the system that is being searched, and how comprehensive or restrictive he or she wants the search to be. The size of the search could be limited somewhat, perhaps to English-language articles, using the following:

respiratory distress syndrome, adult [mesh] AND english [lang].

If the searcher wants to retrieve records that have not been indexed with MeSH or that might have been inconsistently indexed, a free-text search can be run on the terms. One should consider carefully, however, how free the free-text search should be. For example, although a title search may retrieve fewer citations than a free-text search, chances are good that these citations are going to be *highly* relevant. With free-text or title searching, combining synonymous terms, including acronyms, with the Boolean operator *OR* might be desired. Parentheses should be used as follows to avoid confusion:

(ards [title] OR respiratory distress syndrome, adult [mesh]) AND english [lang].

This is a rather simple example of mixing different search elements to maximize the effectiveness of a search (see "Recall and Precision" below). Searching is generally an iterative process; if one strategy does not work, try another.

Additional Indexing Features

Check tag, age group, and publication type search limits generally apply to records that have been indexed. Attempts to use these search limits on PubMed's *in process* and *supplied by publisher* records or within Ovid's Pre-MEDLINE database typically generate zero results.

Sometimes these search limits can be approximated by using free-text search terms to retrieve *unindexed* records. For example, to represent the concept of "review article," the following simple search could be run:

(ards [title] OR adult respiratory distress [title]) AND (review [title] OR overview [title] OR current [title]).

Then searcher could then run a supplemental search designed to retrieve *indexed* records (the field tag [ptyp] means publication type):

respiratory distress syndrome, adult [mesh] AND review [ptyp].

After the two sets have been combined with the Boolean operator *OR*, the individual could add a language limit (e.g., English [language limits should work with both indexed and unindexed records]).

Recall and Precision

The overall effectiveness of a search is usually described in terms of recall and precision. *Recall* is the ratio of relevant records that were retrieved to the number of relevant records in the database. *Precision* is the ratio of relevant records retrieved to the total records retrieved (relevant or irrelevant).

The following example, although somewhat extreme, illustrates the trade offs MEDLINE searchers make between recall and precision. Dr. Sharon Smith, a rheumatologist, is writing a review article on current trends in the use of nonsteroidal antiinflammatory drugs (NSAIDs) in the treatment of rheumatoid arthritis. She starts with the following MEDLINE search strategy: *rheumatoid arthritis AND drug therapy*. Bad move! The search retrieved over 16,000 citations. Although these results probably include most of the MEDLINE citations on NSAIDs and rheumatoid arthritis, she will have to sort through thousands of citations that look at other forms of drug therapy to find the ones she wants.

The good news is that the recall for this search is close to 100%; in other words, Dr. Smith probably retrieved most, if not all, of the citations on NSAIDs and rheumatoid arthritis. The bad news is that the precision of the search is abysmal as the relevant citations are buried in a vast sea of irrelevant citations. Replacing *drug therapy* with *nonsteroidal antiinflammatory drugs* would undoubtedly improve the precision of the search.

Conversely, searchers are often frustrated by low recall, such as when searches retrieve too few citations or none at all. Often, in these cases, the search strategies contained either too many search terms or infrequently used search terms. To improve recall, they should consider using broader terms (e.g., *fruit* rather than *tangerine*) or variant terminology (e.g., if *functional mr imaging* produces few results, try *functional magnetic resonance imaging, fmri,* or *functional mri*).

SIX SEARCH STRATEGIES

The following section provides a quick summary of some search strategies that are discussed in greater detail later in this text. Some strategies take advantage of special features offered by PubMed or Ovid, whereas others are more generic and apply to both systems.

1. Related Articles

Ease of use: High
When to use it: A couple of good articles are needed; one has little time

Searchers interested in ease of use should try PubMed's Related Articles. The Related Articles link retrieves a precalculated set of citations that are similar to or related to the original citation. It may not retrieve everything on a topic, but it is easy to use and it lists the most relevant citations first. (Related Articles is described in more detail in the chapter on PubMed.)

2. Clinical Queries

Ease of use: High
When to use it: A couple of good articles are needed; and one has little time

This strategy can be used in PubMed to emphasize a particular research method in articles on Therapy, Prognosis, Etiology, or Diagnosis. Clinical Queries can also be used to limit the search to "systematic reviews." (Clinical Queries is described in more detail in Chapter 3.)

3. Title Search

Ease of use: High
When to use it: A couple of good articles are needed (a) to display or print, (b) to plug into PubMed's Related Article feature, or (c) to serve as the basis of a more complex search

A title search is one of the most versatile but also one of the most underused MEDLINE search strategies. If the searcher is in a hurry and he or she needs only a couple of highly relevant articles, the individual should consider using a title search. If one is searching for articles about management of the acute abdomen, for example, the search would be *management AND acute AND abdomen* and it would be limited to Title. The advantages of this strategy are many as (a) the user will be able to determine immediately whether the records retrieved are relevant (as opposed to free-text searches, where terms could be scattered through the title, abstract, and so on); (b) the citations can be used as building blocks for subsequent, more complex, more comprehensive searches; and (c) this allows one to retrieve records that lack MeSH or that have been inconsistently indexed.

4. Medical Subject Headings

Ease of use: Moderate
When to use it: Comprehensive searches

The benefits of MeSH searching were described earlier.

5. Medical Subject Headings Plus Title (or Free-Text) Searching

Ease of use: Moderate
When to use it: A good choice for comprehensive searches. A supplemental title search may retrieve unindexed or inconsistently indexed citations without overwhelming the user with large numbers of citations. If the title search retrieves too few citations, the retrieval can always be expanded with a free-text search

The MeSH + Title Search is often the author's strategy of choice because it tends to strike a balance between recall and precision.

6. Multiple Databases

Ease of use: Can be difficult.
When to use it: A means of (a) conducting ultracomprehensive searches (e.g., metaanalyses); (b) researching topics that involve multiple disciplines—a search on the biomechanical properties of hip prostheses could include engineering, medical, and even patent databases; (c) finding information in other databases if a MEDLINE search is unsuccessful

If the searcher wants to maximize recall, then he or she should consider searching multiple databases (and maybe even book catalogs). The searcher's best friend in these cases is often the local medical librarian. Medical librarians can quickly identify the databases or catalogs that best fit the search topic. They can also help devise effective search strategies and can suggest alternatives if the search results prove disappointing.

When searching different databases, the user must remember that different databases (MEDLINE, PsycINFO, BIOSIS, and EMBASE) often use different subject vocabularies. This is particularly important when using a system such as Ovid that allows simultaneous searches of multiple databases. A MeSH term that works for MEDLINE might not be appropriate for BIOSIS.

PUBMED VERSUS OVID

PubMed and Ovid are terrific systems, and both offer an impressive array of powerful search tools and features. If a user has access to Ovid, he or she can take advantage of the best of both systems because PubMed is free. This is the happy situation at Lane Medical Library at Stanford University, where the medical librarians alternate between PubMed and Ovid, choosing one or the other depending on which system is best suited to a particular search.

If new to MEDLINE and perhaps to database searching in general, Ovid (if available) is a great place to start. The Ovid search interface takes advantage of some of MEDLINE's most potent tools—MeSH and subheadings—in a way that is clear and intuitive.

PubMed, on the other hand, tends to shield the searcher from the messy mechanics of some of its search modes. Related Articles, Clinical Queries, and even automatic term mapping happen "under the hood." To the informed, PubMed offers some powerful tools; to the neophyte, the results of a search can be confusing and deceptive.

Following is a brief list of some of the major advantages of both PubMed and Ovid. Subsequent chapters on PubMed and Ovid include more details.

PubMed Advantages

- Fast
- Free
- Growing number of links from PubMed citations to online resources (e.g., electronic journals)
- Multiple search modes
- Multiple document delivery options
- Ability to store searches

Ovid Advantages

- Extremely well-designed search interface
- Multiple-database searching (with duplicate deletion)
- Excellent phrase and adjacency search options
- Ability to rerun saved searches automatically and to receive results via e-mail

BEFORE STARTING TO SEARCH

Before starting a search, the user should consider the following questions.

Is This the Right Place?

This may seem obvious, but the first question one should always ask is, "Is this truly the best resource for answering the question?" Leaping directly into MEDLINE is easy to do whenever one is looking for medical information, but this is not always the best place to be. Looking for the adverse effects of a drug? Try a drug reference book or an electronic resource like ePocrates. Looking for articles on a cancer-related topic? Try CANCERLIT. Not sure where to start? Contact a medical librarian.

How Familiar Is the System?

Again, this might sound obvious, but the more that the searcher knows about the resource, its content, how it is indexed, and how its search interface works, the better equipped he or she will be to search it. The sight of library patrons grumbling when, after a half hour of fruitless searching, they discover that the library's online book catalog is NOT an article database is not uncommon. The searcher should be sure to scan the online help screens or any accompanying print documentation. This is an investment as, ultimately, the user will *save* time, not lose it.

How Are Effective Search Strategies Created?

One of the goals of this handbook is to describe MEDLINE search strategies and how to apply them in PubMed and Ovid MEDLINE. Not knowing when to use MeSH, when to use free-text searching, or when to use both puts the searcher at a distinct disadvantage.

Map the Search

Separate the elements of the search, and think about how they relate to the resource's search tools. Looking for review articles on pharmacologic therapy for atopic dermatitis? Link the MeSH term *dermatitis, atopic* to the subheading Drug Therapy and then limit the search to the publication type *Review*.

Do Not Give Up If One Strategy Fails

Because searching is often an iterative process, try different strategies if the first does not work.

Has Everything On the Topic Been Retrieved?

In a database the size of MEDLINE (currently more than 11 million records), the searcher can never be sure that he or she has retrieved everything.

When in Doubt, Contact a Medical Librarian

When in doubt about a search, contact the local medical librarian.

REFERENCES

1. MEDLINE Fact Sheet. Available at: http://www.nlm.nih.gov/pubs/fact-sheets-medline.html. Accessed June 2002.
2. Funk ME, Reid CA. Indexing consistency in MEDLINE. *Bulletin of the Medical Library Association* 1983;71:176–183.

CHAPTER 3

PubMed

Overview, Screens, and Tools

OVERVIEW OF PUBMED

Launched in 1997 by the National Center for Biotechnology Information (NCBI), a division of the National Library of Medicine (NLM), PubMed (http://www.pubmed.gov/) was one of the first information systems to provide free World Wide Web access to MEDLINE. Integrated within a larger molecular biology retrieval system called Entrez, the initial interface seemed oriented toward researchers in molecular biology and genetics. Gradually, however, as increasing numbers of physicians and other health professionals began to explore the capabilities of PubMed and to provide feedback to the developers, new features were added that dramatically broadened the system's appeal.

Content

PubMed is *not* synonymous with MEDLINE. Although MEDLINE records from 1966 to the present constitute the largest part of PubMed, additional records whose "status" is somewhat different supplement the MEDLINE records.

For example, in PubMed, *in-process* identifies records that are awaiting indexing with Medical Subject Headings (MeSH) and other "value-added" indexing information (e.g., publication types and age groups). Basic bibliographic data for these records (e.g., author, title, abstract) are available for searching, however. Once these records are fully indexed, they will be added to MEDLINE with the notation *indexed for MEDLINE*.

PubMed also contains *supplied by publisher* records—that is, records transmitted to the NLM electronically by journal publishers. Most, but not all, of these eventually receive full indexing. Citations that will not receive full indexing include the following: (a) out-of-scope articles (e.g., on geology, paleontology) from *selectively indexed* MEDLINE journals, and (b) publisher-supplied records from unindexed back issues of journals (e.g., issues published before the acceptance of that journal for inclusion in MEDLINE).

Currently, the NLM is engaged in a significant, far-reaching reorganization of its bibliographic data. The data are clustered into three groups as follows: (a) journal and journal-like records, most of which will be added to PubMed; (b) monographic records (available through LOCATORplus); and (c) journal records from OLDMEDLINE and meeting abstracts (both of which are searchable through the NLM Gateway). OLDMEDLINE is particularly valuable because its coverage extends from 1957 through 1965 (see "Other Databases and Resources" in Appendix 2).

The implications of the reorganization are significant because journal citations from many of NLM's stand-alone databases, including BIOETHICS-

LINE, AIDSLINE, HISTLINE, POPLINE, and SPACELINE, are being added to MEDLINE. Monographic data from these databases are added to LOCATORplus. Meeting abstracts will be accessible through the NLM Gateway.

Links to Other Resources

In addition to the standard bibliographic and indexing data, PubMed supplements its records with links to other online resources. A key component of this service is something called LinkOut, which allows publishers, resource aggregators, and libraries to link Web-based online resources to PubMed citations. For example, a single PubMed record could contain a link to a full-text article, a molecular biology database, portions of several textbooks, and a document delivery service. This linkage between resources is a key element of PubMed (and the entire Entrez system) and one more reason for PubMed's growing popularity.

Keeping up with Changes to PubMed

PubMed's content and search interface are extremely dynamic. To stay informed, the user should regularly check the PubMed New/Noteworthy link. The information about new features is accurate, succinct, and ultracurrent. In addition, PubMed provides extensive information on making the most of its various features under Help, Frequently Asked Questions (FAQ), and Tutorial.

ADVANTAGES AND DISADVANTAGES OF PUBMED

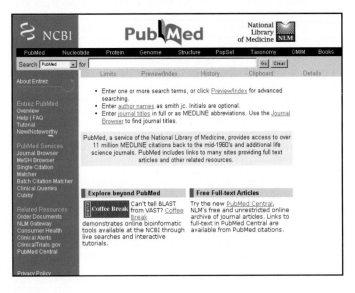

Address	http://pubmed.gov/
Advantages	Fast, free, up to date; multiple search modes; links to a wide array of online resources; searches stored and updated as needed.
Disadvantages	Multiple search modes cause confusion; MeSH browser is underpowered; phrase searching and truncation limited.

MAIN PAGE HIGHLIGHTS

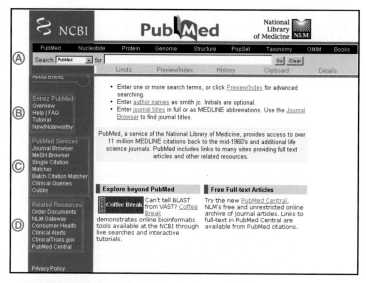

Query Box and Features Bar (A)

Databases and Books. The menu bar provides access to several NCBI resources, as well as links to PubMed's Bookshelf, a collection of searchable online biomedical books; they are also available as a pull-down menu next to Search.

Query Box. Type in the search terms and click the Go button (see "Strategy 1: Query Box" below for more details).

Limits. This is a great way to narrow the search; limits include publication types (e.g., review articles), languages, age groups, and so on.

Preview/Index. Previews displays the number of retrieved citations in a search set before providing them. Index allows searchers to browse lists of search terms and phrases.

History. History keeps track of searches and allows the user to combine them in various ways.

Clipboard. Citations can be saved and printed or downloaded later.

Details. This area shows how the search was translated by PubMed.

Entrez PubMed (B)

Information and news about PubMed and its features are provided here.
Tutorial. This is a Web-based online PubMed tutorial.

PubMed Services (C)

Journal Browser. The journal browser can be used to retrieve citations from a particular journal. It also provides basic information about the journal (e.g., MEDLINE title abbreviation, International Standard Serial Number [ISSN]) and a list of journals with links to full-text Web sites.

MeSH Browser. The PubMed MeSH browser provides a number of features designed to aid searchers in building searches with NLM's MeSH. Enter a term, and the browser will attempt to map it to MeSH (e.g., *wet lung* gets mapped to *pulmonary edema*). The searcher can refine the search by linking the MeSH term to subheadings (e.g., Pulmonary Edema/Prevention and Control). The browser also includes an option for restricting a MeSH search to citations in which the MeSH term has been identified as a major topic.

Unfortunately, the browser is a bit underpowered when it comes to mapping search terms to appropriate MeSH terms (NLM plans to improve the MeSH browser in 2002). *Gi bleeding*, for example, fails to elicit the MeSH *gastrointestinal hemorrhage*. The main reason appears to be that the powerful automatic term mapping feature that plays a vital role in most unqualified query box searches is not connected to the MeSH browser.

So what can the user do? If the MeSH browser fails to provide a reasonable MeSH term, he or she can run a query box search using the Details button to see whether the terms were translated to MeSH (see "Strategy 1: Query Box"). Another approach, known as *bootstrapping*, consists of locating a couple of relevant citations (e.g., with a Title Word or Text Word search), displaying the citations' MeSH terms, and then plugging the relevant MeSH terms into the MeSH browser (see "Strategy 5: MeSH").

Single Citation Matcher. This is a terrific tool for locating a particular citation quickly.

Batch Citation Matcher. This feature is rarely used by the average searcher as it is designed primarily for publishers who want to match online references (e.g., in the bibliography of an online article) to PubMed records.

Clinical Queries. This clinical filter allows searchers to combine a particular disorder with either Therapy, Etiology, Diagnosis, or Prognosis. Research methodology terms (e.g., randomized controlled trials, double-blind studies) are important aspects of the filter. A recent addition to Clinical Queries is an option for limiting searches to Systematic Reviews.

Cubby. Cubby stores searches, allows the user to specify which LinkOut providers are to be displayed in PubMed, and also provides a listing of document delivery providers.

Related Resources (D)

Order Documents. Information can be ordered on Loansome Doc, a document delivery service.

NLM Gateway. This is a Web-based search portal of multiple NLM online databases and catalogs.

Consumer Health. This link to MEDLINEplus includes information on diseases and conditions, links to consumer health information from the National Institutes of Health (NIH), lists of hospitals and physicians, clinical trials, and more.

Clinical Alerts. According to its Web page, Clinical Alerts is designed to "expedite the release of findings from NIH-funded clinical trials where such release could significantly affect morbidity and mortality" (1).

Clinicaltrials.gov. This resource provides consumers and patients with information on clinical research studies.

PubMed Central (PMC). This is a repository of free life sciences journal literature. A "Free in PMC" link on a PubMed citation means that the article is available online through PubMed Central. By clicking the link, a user should be able to retrieve the full text.

DISPLAYING CITATIONS

Displayed Citation List

After running a search in PubMed, typically the user sees a list of citations displayed in the compact Summary format with a collection of links, buttons, and pull-down menus. The citations are listed in the order in which they were *added* to PubMed, with most recent first (use the Sort pull-down menu to redisplay by date of *publication*). These features give the user the option of redisplaying citations in various formats, saving the citations to a file, adding them to a virtual clipboard, and so on. More detailed explanations of these features are included in the following list:

Display Button. Use the display button to redisplay citations after changing the display pull-down menu to a different format.

Display Format Pull-Down Menu. Change the display format from Summary to any one of a wide range of display formats (e.g., Abstract, Citation).

Sort. Sort citations by author, journal name, or publication date. For example, choose Pub Date as the sort order and click the Display button.

Save. Save the citations as a file to the hard drive or a disk.

Text. View citations in a plain text format—no buttons, side bars, or other graphical elements. This is a real paper saver when printing.

Clip Add. Save citations to a Clipboard during a search.

Order. This links to a variety of document delivery services (see "Storing Searches Using the Cubby" for information about choosing a document delivery service).

Show. The Show pull-down menu allows the user to change the number of citations displayed per page.

Changing the Display Format

The Display pull-down menu provides more than a dozen ways to display citations, ranging from XML to Abstract. To change the display, select a format from the Display pull-down menu, then click the Display button. The following four formats are particularly popular:

Summary. This format is the PubMed default display format; it is a good choice for searchers who want to browse a list of citations quickly. Clicking the author's name(s) will display the article's abstract (if one is available).

Abstract. The most common format for downloading and printing. It has the added advantage of displaying publisher and provider icons, some of which link to the full text of journal articles.

MEDLINE. Before importing PubMed citations into a citation management program like EndNote, Reference Manager, or ProCite, the user ***must*** download the citations in the MEDLINE format. These programs need field abbreviations (e.g., AU, author; TI, title) to import the citations properly (see "Citation Management Software").

Citation. Use this indispensable format to display a citation's MeSH terms. If the MeSH terms do not appear, this is because the citation is still classified as *in process* or *supplied by publisher*. Like the Abstract display, this choice also shows publisher and provider icons.

Example: Displaying in the Citation Format

Choose Citation (**A**) from the Display pull-down menu. Click Display (**B**).

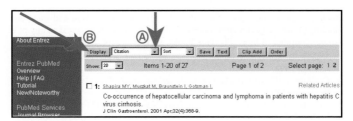

Note that the Citation format displays MeSH and subheadings. Locating a couple of highly relevant citations and then identifying the citations' MeSH terms is one way to locate medical subject headings.

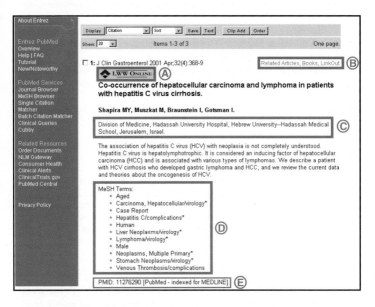

Other Display Features

The preceding citation contains several buttons and links that connect to some interesting online resources, including the following:

Icon Links. The LWW Online link (**A**) implies that the full-text of this article is available online through a Lippincott Williams & Wilkins website. A subscription or fee is often, although not always, required to access full-text articles.

Related Articles. The Related Articles link (**B**) retrieves a precalculated set of citations that are similar to or related to the original citation (for more information, see "Strategy 2: Related Articles").

Books. Clicking the Books link (**B**) will redisplay the citation and may, depending on the subject matter, display links from the abstract's text to any of a growing number of biomedical textbooks, such as the following:

1. Alberts B. *Molecular biology of the cell*, 3rd ed. New York: Garland Publishing, 1994.
2. Griffiths AJF. *An introduction to genetic analysis*, 7th ed. New York: WH Freeman, 2000.
3. Griffiths AJF. *Modern genetic analysis.* New York: WH Freeman, 1999.
4. Lodish HF. *Molecular cell biology*, 4th ed. New York: WH Freeman, 2000.
5. Riddle DL. *C. elegans II.* Plainview, NY: Cold Spring Harbor Laboratory Press, 1997.
6. Varmus H, Coffin JM, Hughes SH. *Retroviruses.* Plainview, NY: Cold Spring Harbor Laboratory Press, 1997.

LinkOut. The LinkOut button (**B**) will display links to those publishers, resource aggregators, and libraries who link Web-based online resources to PubMed citations.

Author Affiliation. This link (**C**) shows the address provided on the article, which is usually that of the first author.

MeSH: Medical Subject Headings. The list of MeSH assigned to this citation (**D**) also shows subheadings, which follow the slash mark, and asterisks (*), which indicate "major topic."

PubMed ID. Each citation contains a unique identifier (**E**) called the PubMed identification (PMID).

BASIC TOOLS

PubMed offers a variety of search tools and features, including Boolean operators (*AND, OR, NOT*), nesting of terms with parentheses, temporary storage for citations via Clipboard, limited truncation, a limited form of phrase searching, and powerful automatic term mapping. For a more general overview of Boolean operators, truncation, nesting, and phrase searching, see Chapter 2.

Automatic Term Mapping

Any unqualified search entered in PubMed's query box is processed using automatic term mapping. This differs from a "qualified" search, in which the searcher might select a particular field or fields to search (e.g., a Title Word search). Search terms are run through a series of tables, lists, and indexes in an elaborate effort to increase the effectiveness of the search. Listed in order of the search, they are as follows:

- MeSH Translation Table
- Journals Translation Table
- Phrase List
- Author Index

The process is often, although not always, surprisingly successful. An explanation of how automapping works follows (2).

First, search terms are compared against the contents of the MeSH Translation Table, which includes MeSHs, subheadings, and so on. For example, *kidney stones* is mapped to the MeSH *kidney calculi*. PubMed then runs a MeSH search of *kidney calculi* and supplements it with a Text Word of the original search term *kidney stones*. The search would appear as follows: *kidney calculi [MeSH Terms] OR kidney stones [Text Word]*. Keep in mind that the supplemental Text Word search is quite broad as it includes titles and abstracts, so it may retrieve more citations than needed.

If the terms are not matched, PubMed moves to the Journal Translation Table. If the search terms are the full journal name, MEDLINE abbreviation, or journal ISSN number, PubMed will retrieve citations from that journal. If the unqualified journal name is also a MeSH term (e.g., *cerebral cortex*), PubMed will *not* search it as a *journal name*. In these cases, use PubMed's Journal Browser or qualify terms with the journal field tag (e.g., *cerebral cortex [journal name]*).

PubMed also searches a limited Phrase List containing several hundred thousand phrases. For example, *renal scan* matches *renal scan* in the Phrase List. The phrase is subsequently run as an All Fields search: *renal scan [All Fields]*. All Fields is just what it implies and is an extremely broad search (see "Phrase Searching") for more information.

If the terms have not yet been matched in the previous tables and lists and the term has one or two letters after it, PubMed will consult an Author Index. If only the first initial is entered, PubMed will automatically truncate the search to account for varying initials. In other words, a search on "o'leary j" would retrieve *o'leary j, o'leary ja, o'leary jm* and so on.

If still no match has been made, PubMed will begin to strip away terms from right to left in a vigorous attempt to find a match. For example, *atrial septum closure* does not match in the aforementioned tables or lists, and so the term *closure* is removed. *Atrial septum*, however, does find a match in the Phrase List, so it is plugged into an All Fields search. *Closure* does not have a match in any of the translation tables, and it will also be plugged into an All Fields search. The two then are combined with *AND*. Clicking the Details button (**A**) shows PubMed's translation of the search terms (**B**):

The automapping process is complicated, but knowing how it works can give a user a better idea of how PubMed approaches the interpretation of unqualified search terms. The searcher should also be sure to use the Details button when running unqualified searches via PubMed's query box to see how the terms were translated (see "Strategy 1: Query Box" for more details)

Boolean Operators

The following things need to be remembered when using Boolean operators in PubMed: (a) *AND* is assumed, so actually typing in the *AND* operator is optional. On occasion, however, PubMed will treat adjacent terms as phrases, so the user should check the search with the Details button to make sure that he or she gets what is expected. The author finds it easier to keep track of what is going on in his searches when he includes *AND*. (b) Put all Boolean operators in upper case (e.g., AND, OR, NOT). (c) Remember that terms are searched from left to right.

Example: Searching Using the Boolean Operator NOT

To locate articles that discuss cluster headache, but *not* migraine, type *cluster headache NOT migraine*. Click Go.

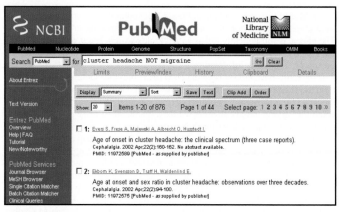

Truncation

In PubMed, the truncation symbol is the asterisk (*). Currently, PubMed will search *only* the first 150 variations of a truncated word (according to NLM, this will soon be increased). For example, a search of *epid** results in the following message: "*Wildcard search for 'epid*' used only the first 150 variations. Lengthen the root word to search for all endings.*" So, the user could then lengthen the root word to *epidemiol**.

Example: Using the Truncation Symbol

A subsequent search on: *epidemiol* AND beriberi AND vitamin** does not evoke the truncation warning message.

Nesting with Parentheses

Parentheses force PubMed to perform operations within the parentheses as a group *before* combining them with terms and operators outside the parentheses. For example, in the following search, *patient compliance AND (sodium restricted diet OR low sodium diet)*, terms within the parentheses are searched first, which overrides the usual search order of processing left to right. These results then are combined with the phrase *patient compliance*. The author often uses parentheses to combine synonymous terms with the *OR* operator (e.g., calcul* OR stone*).

Example: Using Parentheses

To locate citations discussing the use of urography in kidney trauma, the user could type *urography AND trauma AND (kidney OR renal)*.

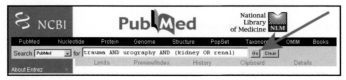

Phrase Searching

PubMed does *not* perform true term adjacency searching. As was described in "Automatic Term Mapping," if a phrase cannot be located in the various tables and lists, including the Phrase List, PubMed will break the phrase into smaller pieces looking for a match. If PubMed fails to find a match, individual terms will be combined using *AND* and searched in All Fields.

If, however, the user encloses the phrase in quotes (e.g., "continuous quality improvement"), PubMed will consult a much larger index containing millions of phrases that have been generated from citation titles, abstracts, MeSH, and so on. If the phrase is located, it will be searched in All Fields. If the phrase is not located, PubMed will ignore the quotation marks and will process the phrase with automatic term mapping.

Example: Phrase Searching Using Quotation Marks

A query box search of *pressure point* initially fails to locate the terms as a phrase, so term mapping breaks the phrase apart and runs a MeSH and Text Word search of *pressure* and an All Fields search of *point*. This is not quite what the user wanted.

Instead, the searcher could put the phrase in quotes. Type *"pressure point,"* click Go, and then click on the Details button (**A**) to see how PubMed translated this search (**B**).

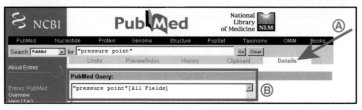

NOTE: Quotation marks around a phrase deactivate automatic term mapping; however, if the phrase is unrecognized in either the Phrase List or index, the quotation marks are ignored and the terms are processed using automatic term mapping. If the phrase in quotes (e.g., *"Esophageal Motility Disorders"*) happens to match an explodable MeSH term (i.e., one with narrower MeSH terms), the narrower MeSH terms (e.g., *gastroesophageal reflux*) will *not* be included in the search. Therefore, one should use quotes with caution.

Clipboard

PubMed allows the storage of up to 500 citations in a temporary space called Clipboard. Later, the user can display, save, or print the stored citations (Clipboard retains the citations for 1 hour). A particularly nice feature of Clipboard is the deletion of duplicate citations.

Example: Saving Citations to the Clipboard

Simply select some citations and click Clip Add.

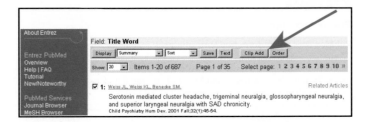

PubMed confirms that the citations were saved to the Clipboard. To retrieve them, click on Clipboard.

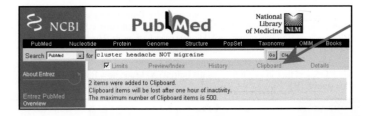

The screen shot below shows the citations saved to Clipboard. Citation numbers of saved citations are highlighted in green. To clear the Clipboard, simply click the Clip Remove button.

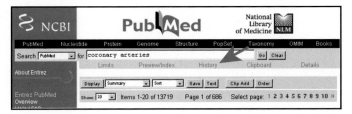

COMBINING SEARCHES

Overview

A user can combine searches in PubMed in several ways. Of course, combining searches in a single search string (e.g., a query box search of *bronchopulmonary dysplasia AND mechanical ventilation*) is one way. Or, one can run searches of the different elements, and the results of these can then be combined in various ways using PubMed's History feature.

Example: Combining Search Sets Using History

A query box search on *coronary arteries* was conducted. The user can narrow the search by combining it with an author search that was conducted earlier by clicking History.

Combine the two sets (**A**) by typing *#1 AND #2* (**B**). Now either click Preview (**C**) to see how many citations would be obtained or click Go (**D**) to run the search and retrieve the citations.

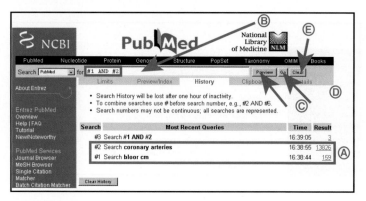

NOTE: History retains up to 100 searches. The Clear History button (**E**) will clear the search histories.

Preview/Index

The Preview/Index screen provides a variety of options for building a search. It has some features that it shares in common with History, but it also has some important differences (e.g., it only retains the last three search queries).

Preview

The first Preview button is located across from the query box; it can be used to view the *number* of citations for a particular query box search. The second Preview button is located in the *Add Term(s) to Query* portion of the screen; it can be used to add terms to the query box *and* to preview the number of search results.

Index

The Index button allows one to scan and select terms from specific search fields. For example, if a user wants to choose a publication type that is not available on the Limits screen, which includes only the most popular publication types (e.g., Review), he or she could choose Publication Type from the Preview/Index pull-down menu (**A**), click the Index button (**B**), and then select the desired publication type from the resulting list (e.g., Historical Article) (**C**).

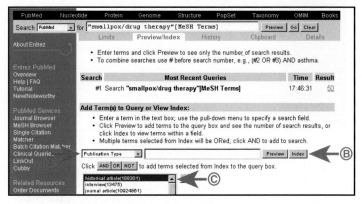

A user can choose more than one term by holding down the control (CTRL) key on a personal computer (PC) or the command key on a Macintosh (Mac) while selecting the terms with the mouse.

AND, OR, and NOT Buttons

These buttons can be used to add terms to the query box, as well as the specified Boolean operator. Type in a term, or use the Index button to select a term(s) from a list and then click the appropriate Boolean operator button. Use the Preview button to preview the results of the search and the Go button to run the search and retrieve the results. Remember that PubMed will process the search from left to right.

LIMITING SEARCHES

Most searchers find that they must apply restrictions, or Limits, to the searches they run in PubMed. Although PubMed's Limits page may not offer access to *every* search limit, it does offer a pull-down menu for some of the more important ones. Clicking Limits will take the user to the Limits screen.

NOTE: Remember that many limits only apply to fully indexed (i.e., MED-LINE) citations. In other words, *in-process* or *supplied by publisher* citations will be lost if the Publication Type, Age Group, Gender, or Human or Animal limits are applied. Language limits can be safely used.

All Fields. This is the default setting of this pull-down menu. The All Fields manu includes the option known as Text Word, which enables free-text searching for multiple fields, including abstracts, MeSH tems, subheadings, personal names as subjects, and MEDLINE Secondary Source.

Publication Types. This pull-down menu allows searchers to restrict the results to documents of a certain format (e.g., clinical trial, editorial, metaanalysis, or practice guidelines).

Ages. PubMed provides an Ages pull-down menu that includes several age groups that combine more specific groups (e.g., All Children includes Newborn, Infant, Preschool Child, Child, and Adolescent).

Human and Animal. This limit restricts the search to human studies, animal studies, or both.

Publication Date. The user can restrict the search by the publication date of the article. Enter only one year (e.g., 1995) in the From box, and PubMed will automatically search 1995 to present.

Entrez Date. Restrict the search by the dates that citations were added to PubMed. Conceivably, one could use this option to retrieve citations added after the last search, although the stored search utility, the Cubby, does essentially the same thing (see "Storing Searches Using the Cubby").

Gender. Choose either male or female.

Subsets. Undoubtedly, new subsets will be added to PubMed as other specialty databases are closed and their journal citations are added to MEDLINE (e.g.,

HISTLINE and SPACELINE). PubMed subsets currently fall into the following three main groups:

1. Citation status

In-process: ultracurrent but not yet indexed (i.e., lacking MeSH terms, subheadings, publication types).

Publisher: electronically submitted to NLM by publishers but not indexed.

MEDLINE: MEDLINE only, fully indexed.

2. Groupings of topically related journals

Core Clinical Journals: restricts to 120 journals that form the core of many small-sized to medium-sized hospital libraries.

Dental Journals: restricts search to dental journals.

Nursing Journals: restricts search to nursing journals.

PubMed Central: consists of an archive of articles whose content is available without charge.

3. Subject groupings based on preformulated search strategies

AIDS: restricts search to citations on AIDS.

Bioethics: restricts to citations on ethics relating to the life sciences.

Complementary Medicine: restricts to articles in the area of complementary and alternative medicine.

Space Life Sciences: restricts to citations in the area of space and the life sciences.

Toxicology: restricts to citations on toxicology.

Example: Limiting a Search

The following example shows a search of *otitis media* limited to English, Core Clinical Journals, Human Studies, 1990 to present, Review Articles, and Children.

NOTE: Be sure to *uncheck* the Limits check box to run another search with different search limits.

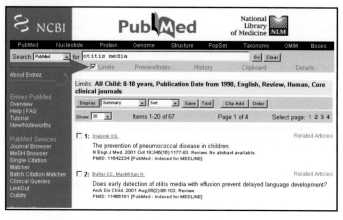

Searching

LOCATING A SINGLE CITATION

PubMed's Single Citation Matcher is the tool to use to locate a citation quickly.

Example: Locating a Single Citation

One of the fastest ways to locate a citation is with the author, first page, and publication year (e.g., author "Smith," page 222, date 1999).

To run the search, click Search.

Obviously, one could use journal names or journal abbreviations, but this may cause trouble unless the journal title is straightforward (e.g., *Journal of the American Medical Association [JAMA]* or *Lancet*). For example, if the abbreviation entered is not a standard MEDLINE abbreviation (e.g., *Bio Med Chem* instead of *Bioorg Med Chem*) or if the user misspells the full journal title (*Bioorganic Medical Chemistry* instead of *Bioorganic Medicinal Chemistry*), PubMed will not be able to locate the citation.

AUTHOR SEARCHING

When performing author searches in PubMed, keep the following in mind: (a) MEDLINE does *not* understand first or middle names, so use initials; (b) sometimes authors use their middle initials and sometimes they do not; (c) if a user is searching for articles *about* a person, add the tag [PS] (personal name as subject) after the person's name (e.g., *shumway ne [PS]*); (d) compound names can be entered without punctuation (e.g., *van der meer r*); and (e) PubMed automatically truncates after a single initial to account for varying middle initials.

An author search in PubMed can be run in one of the following ways: an unqualified search in the search query box, a qualified search using the author field tag [au], or Author Field from the Limits screen.

Using the Query Box

Type in the author's last name and first and middle initials.

Example: Author Search in the Query Box

To locate articles by Colin M. Bloor, type *bloor cm*. Click Go.

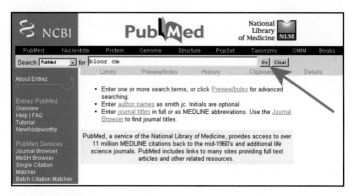

Example: Author Search When the Middle Initial Is Unknown

What if the user does not know the middle initial? In that case, simply search with first initial. PubMed will retrieve citations with the last name, first initial, *any* middle initial, or no middle initial at all.

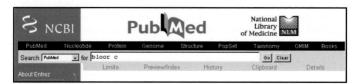

Using the Author Field Tag

If the user does not know any initials, he or she should search the author field directly; otherwise, PubMed may look for the last name in any field (e.g., a search on *Hopkins* will retrieve citations containing *Johns Hopkins* in the Affiliation field). One way to do this is with the author field tag *[au]*.

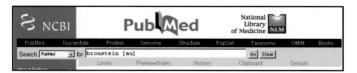

NOTE: If *only* the last name and first initial are wanted, put the name in quotes followed by the author field tag (e.g., *"smith j" [au]*).

Using the All Fields Pull-Down Menu

If the user has forgotten the field tag for author, he or she can go to Limits and select Author Name from the All Fields pull-down menu.

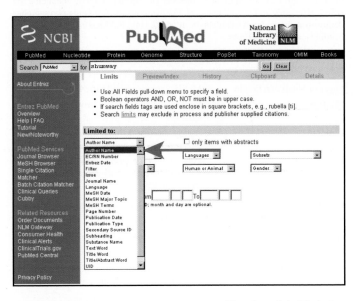

NOTE: Remember that the limits the user sets will apply until the Limits box is unchecked.

TOPIC SEARCHING

Overview

PubMed undeniably provides the discriminating searcher with an impressive array of powerful tools. From the deceptively bland query box to the the sophisticated Related Articles, PubMed offers a collection of search options that few other MEDLINE systems can match. However, a bit of practice is needed to know which of these options works best for a particular search.

Integrating the Search into PubMed

PubMed can accommodate a wide range of search strategies. A solid grasp of PubMed's features and search modes gives the searcher the ability to integrate the search more closely into the framework of PubMed, thereby enhancing the search efficiency and overall retrieval. For example, the following two searches demonstrate how search terms can be integrated into PubMed using MeSH, subheadings, and search limits.

Example 1. A user is searching for review articles on the etiology of fevers of unknown origin in children.

Fever of Unknown Origin	MeSH term (use MeSH Browser)
Etiology	Subheading (use MeSH Browser or Clinical Queries)
Children	Age group (use Limits, then go to the Ages pull-down menu, and select All Child)
Review articles	Publication type (use Limits, then go to the Publication Types pull-down menu, and select Review)

Example 2. The searcher is looking for some *epidemiologic* studies on *atopic dermatitis* from some *core clinical journals*.

Atopic Dermatitis	MeSH term (use MeSH Browser)
Epidemiology	Subheading (use MeSH Browser)
Core Clinical Journals	Subset (go to Limits, then use the Subset pull-down menu, and select Core Clinical Journals)

NOTE: Trying to figure out which part of the search goes where can be tricky. One shortcut is locating a couple of relevant citations, redisplaying them in the Citation format to see how they have been indexed, and then plugging in the indexing terms (see "Strategy 5: Medical Subject Headings").

Developing a Search Strategy

A searcher's choice of a particular MEDLINE search strategy usually involves the following three factors: (a) knowledge of the search system; (b) time available for searching; and (c) required depth, or inclusiveness, of the search (see Chapter 2, "Elements of an Effective Search"). For example, if a hurried searcher needs to locate a few articles on the treatment of meconium aspiration, he or she could select PubMed's Clinical Queries, enter *meconium aspiration*, and click Search. This approach is simple and fast, and, in this case, it retrieves a reasonably small set of relevant citations.

On the other hand, if one has several months to write a review article on gestational diabetes, he or she could run a more complex MeSH plus free-text search that strongly emphasizes retrieval. The search might be fairly complicated, and it could take some time to create, but the chances are greater that the search will retrieve a high percentage of the journal literature on the subject.

The five distinct search strategies discussed below have been chosen because they adapt easily to the ever-fluctuating variables of skill, time, and inclusiveness. Each strategy includes commentary on when to use it, when to be careful, how it works, and sample search examples using screen shots. The strategies are listed *roughly* in order of ease of use.

Strategy 1: Query Box

Strategy 2: Related Articles

Strategy 3: Clinical Query

Strategy 4: Title Search

Strategy 5: MeSH Browser

Search Strategy 1: Query Box

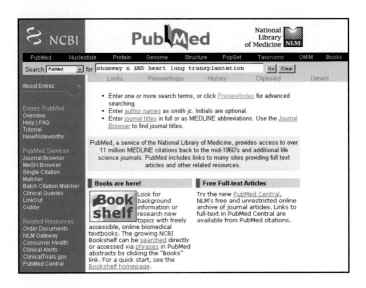

Advantages

Fast! It uses PubMed's automatic term mapping to retrieve, among other things, MeSH terms.

Disadvantages

It tends to retrieve large quantities of citations, and it often is less precise than other strategies. Unqualified search terms are sometimes translated in unexpected ways.

When To Use

It is surprisingly effective for simple searches combining easily defined topics (e.g., *fiber AND colorectal cancer*), and it is particularly appealing to the hurried searcher who lacks the time to learn the finer points of PubMed searching.

When To Be Careful

Automatic term mapping lies at the heart of the unqualified query box search. (See "Automatic Term Mapping" for more information.) It is powerful, but, depending on how term mapping parses the search, it often retrieves more citations than the user wanted. For example, terms that are matched to MeSH are also run as supplemental Text Word searches. Because a Text Word search includes titles, abstracts, and so on, the searcher could end up sorting through large numbers of irrelevant citations.

In addition, if a term is matched to a subheading (e.g., Surgery, Drug Therapy, Prevention and Control, Etiology), the subheading is *not* linked directly to a specific MeSH term but it instead is *free floating*. Thus, a search on *surgery AND coronary disease* retrieves not only citations about surgical management of coronary artery disease but also citations on the surgical management of *prostate cancer* in someone *with* coronary artery disease. In other words, the subheading *surgery* attaches to *any* MeSH term in the citation (in this case, *prostate neoplasms*), not necessarily to *coronary disease*. For more precision, the user can use the MeSH Browser to link a subheading *directly* to a MeSH term (see "Strategy 5: Medical Subject Headings").

Occasionally, term mapping can add terms the user does not want. For example, *audiovisual teaching aids* maps to the MeSH term *acquired immunodeficiency syndrome*. This usually is not a big problem, but it is one reason to use the Details link to ensure that the search has been translated as intended.

In the author's experience, even though the search results may include a significant percentage of the PubMed citations on a particular topic (high recall), a lot of time might still need to be spent in sifting through the results to find them.

How It Works

See "Automatic Term Mapping" for more information.

Keep In Mind

This strategy is fast but often at a price. Use the Details button to make sure that the search is translated properly.

Query Box Examples

Example 1: A search that combines two simple topics. To locate articles that describe the effects of vitamin C on the common cold, type *vitamin C AND common cold* and then click the Go button.

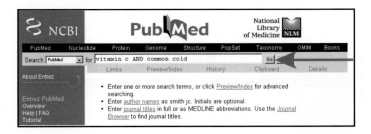

Clicking the Details link (**A**) reveals how the search was translated (**B**).

Vitamin C was mapped to the MeSH term *ascorbic acid*, and *common cold* was mapped to the MeSH term *common cold*. PubMed performed an additional Text Word search of the initial search terms to enhance retrieval.

NOTE: One can edit any of the search terms displayed in the PubMed Query window. Once editing is complete, simply click on the Search button to rerun the search. Clicking on the URL button embeds the search terms in a URL, which the user can then bookmark with the Web browser.

One can restrict the size of a search set by applying some search limits. Clicking Limits (**A**) pulls up the Limits screen. To limit the search to English-language articles from 1990 to the present, simply select English from the Language pull-down menu, and put 1990 in the From box to the right of Publication Date. Once the limits are selected (**B**), clicking Go (**C**) applies the limits to the search.

To store the first two citations temporarily, select them by clicking in their checkboxes (**D**), and then click the Clip Add button (**E**). When the search in PubMed is complete, one can display, print, save, or order the stored citations by clicking on Clipboard (**F**).

Example 2: Combine two or more topics. To locate articles that discuss quality of life after heart transplantation in children, start by unchecking the Limits checkbox (**A**) and type *quality of life AND heart transplantation*; then click Go (**B**).

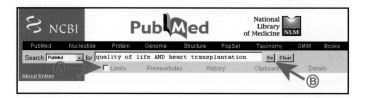

Clicking the Details link (**C**) shows what went on "under the hood." In this case, PubMed again mapped to the appropriate MeSH terms. Next, click Limits (**D**).

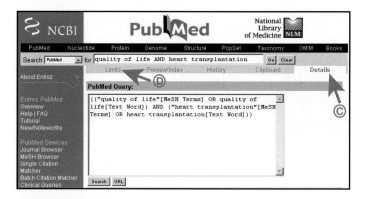

Select All Child, Human, and English, and enter a publication date of 1995 to present. Click Go.

PubMed	Nucleotide	Protein	Genome	Structure	PopSet	Taxonomy	OMIM	Books

Search PubMed for quality of life AND heart transplantation   Go Clear

Limits   Preview/Index   History   Clipboard   Details

About Entrez

Entrez PubMed
Overview
Help | FAQ
Tutorial
New/Noteworthy

- Use All Fields pull-down menu to specify a field.
- Boolean operators AND, OR, NOT must be in upper case.
- If search fields tags are used enclose in square brackets, e.g., rubella [ti].
- Search limits may exclude in process and publisher supplied citations.

Limited to:

PubMed Services
Journal Browser
MeSH Browser
Single Citation
Matcher
Batch Citation Matcher
Clinical Queries
Cubby

All Fields ▼		☐ only items with abstracts	
Publication Types ▼	English ▼	Subsets ▼
All Child: 0-18 years ▼	Human ▼	Gender ▼
Entrez Date ▼		

Publication Date ▼ From 1995 [ ] To [ ] [ ]
Use the format YYYY/MM/DD; month and day are optional.

Again, use Clip Add to save the citations to the Clipboard.

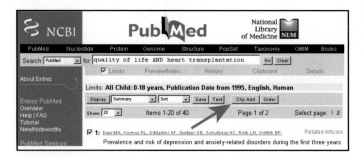

Example 3: Combining a search with earlier searches. One can combine a search with earlier searches using History, an approach described earlier in "Combining Searches."

Enter the search terms *rheumatoid arthritis AND prednisone* and then click Go.

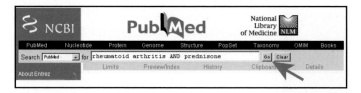

To combine the results with an earlier search on the etiology of osteoporosis, click History.

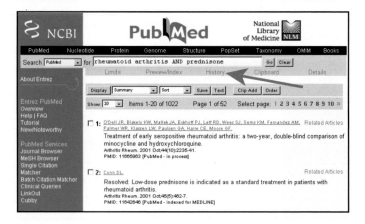

Type *AND #2* (**A**) to the end of the search statement and click Go (**B**).

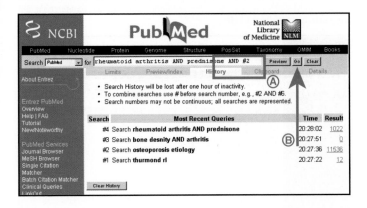

At this point, the user could click Limits to add search limits, such as language, date range, and so on.

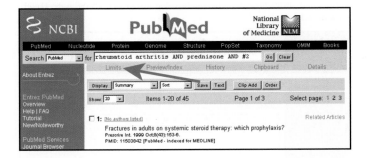

Example 4: Limitations of the Query Box. The query box is not omniscient. To locate articles on the impact of cold temperatures on ischemic heart disease, type *cold AND ischemic heart disease*. Click Go.

If the searcher clicks Details (**A**), the results might be surprising. PubMed correctly mapped *cold* (as in the temperature) to the appropriate MeSH term *cold* but also to MeSH terms that the user would not want, such as *common cold* and *lung diseases, obstructive* (**B**).

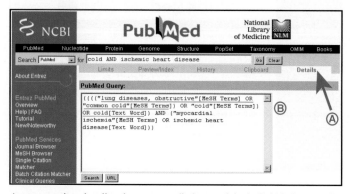

As was mentioned earlier, the user can edit the search in the PubMed query window. As the next screen shot illustrates, the MeSH terms *common cold* and *lung diseases, obstructive* were removed, as was the Text Word search of *cold* (*cold* in titles and abstracts seems a bit too broad at this point). To rerun the search, click Search.

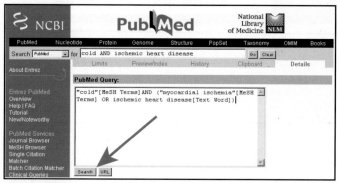

After restricting the search to English, Human, and 1990 to present, some highly relevant citations are revealed.

ClinicalTrials.gov
PubMed Central

☐ **4:** Cabrera K, Schwartz RW.   Related Articles

Privacy Policy

Ulcerative colitis: natural history and medical management.
Curr Surg. 2001 Mar;58(2):195-197. No abstract available.
PMID: 11275244 [PubMed - as supplied by published]

☐ **5:** Marion JF.   Related Articles

The medical management of acute and chronic ulcerative colitis.
Acta Gastroenterol Belg. 2000 Jul-Sep;63(3):294-8. Review.
PMID: 11189989 [PubMed - indexed for MEDLINE]

☐ **6:** Belaiche J, Louis E.   Related Articles

Initial medical management of severe acute ulcerative colitis.
Acta Gastroenterol Belg. 2000 Jul-Sep;63(3):275-8.
PMID: 11189987 [PubMed - indexed for MEDLINE]

Search Strategy 2: Related Articles

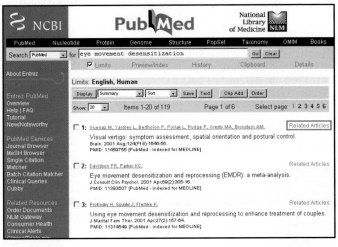

Advantages

It is extremely fast; it can retrieve citations that other strategies might miss.

Disadvantages

Citations with abstracts tend to generate results that also contain abstracts; citations without abstracts generally produce results without abstracts (NLM is attempting to improve this aspect of the algorithm). It is not a comprehensive search strategy, so one should supplement it with other strategies to increase recall (see "Strategy 5: Medical Subject Headings"). It also drops any search limits one might have applied. Relevancy can drop off rapidly.

When to Use

It is good for retrieving a few highly relevant citations quickly, and it can be extremely effective as an adjunct to other search strategies, particularly if the initial retrieval set is low.

When to Be Careful

This strategy is not terribly effective for comprehensive searches. Relevancy often drops off sharply after the first 20 to 30 citations. Any limits the user applies in the initial search (e.g., language or publication date) will be lost when using Related Articles. One can, however, reapply them later, although at the risk of losing relevant citations (see "Related Articles Example" below). Also, one must find a relevant citation before it can be used.

How It Works

Related Articles uses a complex algorithm to identify a particular citation's related citations. The best matches are saved and stored in a precalculated set. Citations that lack the Related Articles link simply have not yet been run through the algorithm. The algorithm is based, among other things, on term frequency and the position of terms within a citation (e.g., a term in the title carries more weight than a term buried in an abstract).

Keep in Mind

Citations retrieved by Related Articles are listed in order of relevance (i.e., the most relevant is listed first). As was mentioned earlier, while scanning through the citations, the user will find that relevancy can drop off rapidly.

Related Articles Example

In a search for English-language articles that discuss cognitive performance and circadian rhythms, a query box search using truncation (*) on *cognitive performance AND circadian rhythm** retrieves 109 citations.

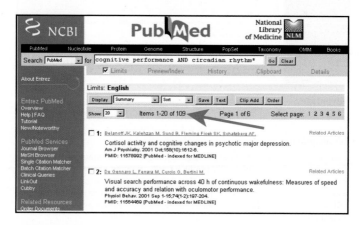

Scrolling through the citations reveals one article of particular interest. Click on the Related Articles link to find others like it.

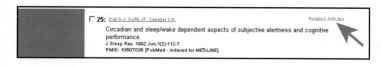

PubMed retrieved 130 citations. While the loss of search limits may not be immediately obvious, the search limit English was dropped. To reapply it, do *not* click on Limits right away; instead, click on History.

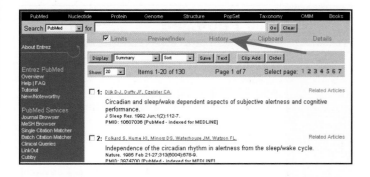

The Related Articles search is represented by the statement, "Related Articles for PubMed (Select 10607036)." The number 10607036 is the unique PubMed ID number for the original citation. Use the Clear button (**A**) to remove the previous search, and then enter the search set number (**#2**) into the Query box (**B**). Click Go (**C**).

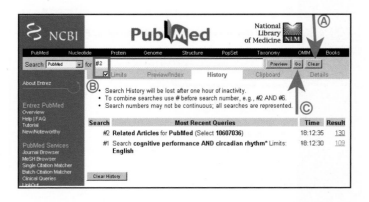

The search limits have been reapplied!

NOTE: Reapply other search limits (e.g., publication types and age groups) with care because some relevant citations may be lost. Also, remember that the citations will no longer be listed in the order of the most relevant first.

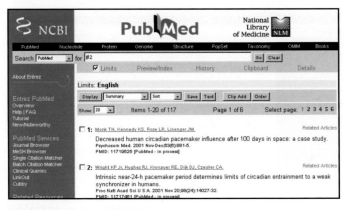

Search Strategy 3: Clinical Queries

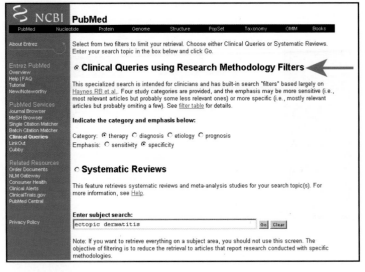

Advantages

It is fast, and the emphasis is on "best evidence."

Disadvantages

It is not comprehensive, nor is it the best choice for certain topics.

When to Use

Use this strategy to emphasize a particular research methodology in articles on either Therapy, Prognosis, Etiology, or Diagnosis. For example, the search "hedge" behind Therapy + Specificity includes the terms *double*, *blind*, *placebo*, and so on.

Use Clinical Queries to limit a search to systematic reviews. According to the PubMed help page, these include citations identified as systematic reviews, metaanalyses, reviews of clinical trials, consensus development conferences, and guidelines. The Clinical Queries screen also contains links to additional explanatory information.

When to Be Careful

Clinical Queries often retrieves either far more or far fewer citations than one might expect, so this strategy should not be used if one is trying to run a carefully constructed, comprehensive search. Also, some search topics simply do not lend themselves to this approach; for example, a search for articles on treatment of gunshot wounds to the chest will not retrieve many articles, no doubt because of the lack of double-blind studies or randomized controlled trials.

How It Works

Type in the name of a disease and then select Treatment, Diagnosis, Prognosis, or Etiology. Further refining the search is possible by selecting Sensitivity (similar to Recall, Sensitivity increases the number of citations retrieved while possibly lowering precision) or Specificity (like Precision, it emphasizes relevance, which means fewer citations to sift through; some citations, however, may be missed). Each search uses a predesigned search hedge consisting of combinations of free-text terms, MeSH, free-floating subheadings (e.g., drug therapy), and so on.

Keep in Mind

The author does not use the Clinical Queries search mode much because it forces the user to accept the underlying, predesigned search hedges. If a searcher wants to have more control over the search construction, he or she may prefer to use other approaches. Before using Clinical Queries, searchers should take a look at the Clinical Queries filter table, which describes how the search hedges are designed.

Clinical Queries Example

To locate articles on the *treatment of atopic dermatitis*, select Therapy (**A**) and Specificity (**B**) and click the Search button (**C**).

57

Even after choosing Specificity, more than 400 citations remain, so use Limits to restrict the search further.

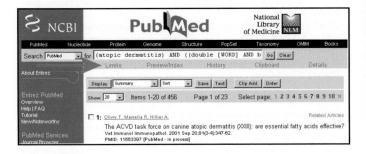

The search was limited to English, Human, and 1995 to present.

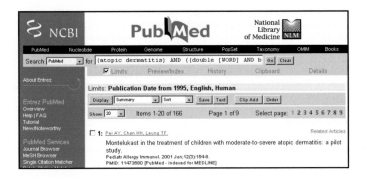

Search Strategy 4: Title Search

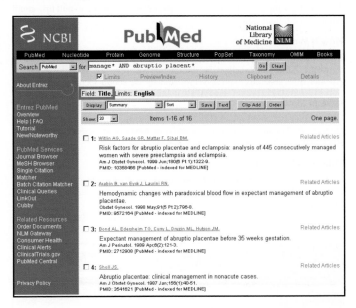

Advantages

It is fast with a high degree of relevance. It can retrieve citations that have not been indexed with MeSH (i.e., citations identified as *in process* or *supplied by* the *publisher*). This is a great starting place for more complex strategies.

Disadvantages

This strategy is definitely not comprehensive.

When to Use

Title searches offer an effective strategy (a personal favorite) for identifying a couple of highly relevant articles quickly. Perhaps more importantly, a well-designed title search is one of the best ways to lay the groundwork for a more sophisticated and comprehensive search (see "Strategy 5: Medical Subject Headings").

HELPFUL HINT: Looking for extremely current overviews of a particular topic? Perhaps interested in citations that are in process and that are not yet indexed with the publication type Review? Try running a title search that combines the search topic and terms like *management*, *review*, *trends*, or *current* (as in *current approaches in . . .*). The following is an example:

> *(manage* [ti] OR review [ti] OR trends [ti] OR current [ti]) AND hepatitis c [ti].*

When to Be Careful

This is not a comprehensive search strategy; rather, it is meant to pull up a small number of citations quickly.

How It Works

In the writer's experience, if an author uses a title that includes the given search terms, the chances are excellent that that citation is *extremely* relevant to the search. After all, titles generally express, very succinctly, the central themes of the article.

Keep in Mind

Using terms that could reasonably be expected to appear in the title of the article (e.g., *PET scans* versus *positron emission tomography scans*) is important. Also, make frequent use of truncation and synonyms.

Title Search Examples

Example 1: Recent articles on the management of ulcerative colitis. To locate a couple of recent articles on the management of ulcerative colitis, first limit the search to English, 1995 to present.

Type *manage* AND ulcerative colitis*. Be sure to click Limits (**A**) *before* running the search.

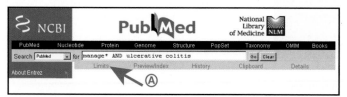

Choose Title (**B**), English (**C**), and 1995 to present (**D**). If any more search limits (e.g., review articles or age groups) are added, *in-process* or *supplied by publisher* citations will be missed. Click Go (**E**).

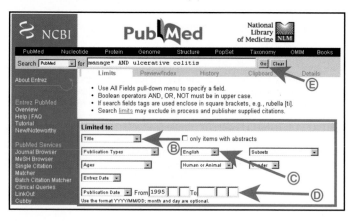

Not bad at all. Some of the citations appear to be quite relevant.

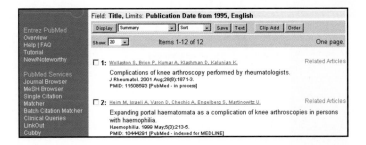

Example 2: Possible complications for knee arthroscopy. A patient inquires about possible *complications* from a planned *arthroscopy of her knee*. Limit the search to Title, English, 1995 to present.

Type *complicat* AND arthroscop* AND knee** into the query box. The limits from the previous search still apply (note the check mark in the little box next to Limits). Click Go.

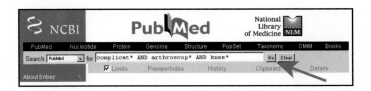

Great. Several of the citations may be on target.

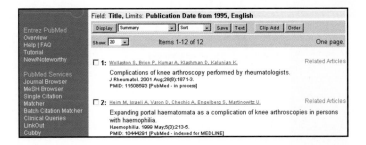

Example 3: Recent articles on ovarian disease in women taking tamoxifen.
Have any articles been written recently that look at *ovarian disease* in women
taking *tamoxifen* to *prevent or treat breast cancer*? Limit to English, 1995 to
present.

Type *tamoxifen AND ovar* AND breast* in the query box. Next, click on the
word Limits (*not* the checkbox).

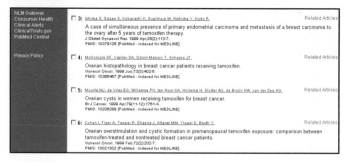

Limit to English language, 1995 to present (**A**). Click Go (**B**).

Many of the citations look relevant.

NOTE: These highly relevant citations can form the core of additional search
strategies, such as those using Related Articles (see "Strategy 2: Related Articles") or MeSH (see "Strategy 5: Medical Subject Headings").

Search Strategy 5: Medical Subject Headings

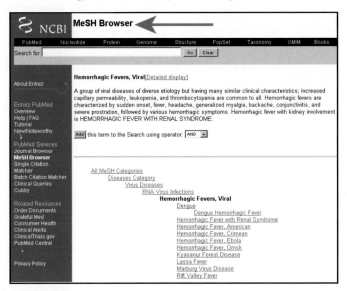

Advantages

Relevance and retrieval are high.

Disadvantages

This can be more complicated, and it may take more time than other strategies. Some citations lack MeSH terms. Inconsistencies in indexing mean that some citations might be missed.

When to Use

This is often the strategy of choice for searches that go beyond, "Give me one or two good citations fast." MeSH headings and subheadings, particularly when used via the MeSH browser, offer the searcher the maximum amount of control over a PubMed search. A supplemental title or free-text search (a title search is usually the author's preference) can retrieve many of the unindexed or inconsistently indexed citations missed by the original MeSH search.

As described in "Strategy 1: Query Box," automatic term mapping often can perform a similar sort of search—that is, mapping terms to MeSH and augmenting the results with a free-text search. Unfortunately, the searches generated by automatic term mapping frequently are less precise than those developed within the MeSH browser (see "Strategy 1: Query Box" for more information). If the query box consistently retrieves too many citations or if it simply lacks the precision that is needed, try using the MeSH browser.

When to Be Careful

This approach can sometimes take longer than other strategies. It requires the user to identify the MeSH terms for the search. One can do this with (a) the MeSH browser, (b) a "bootstrapping" title search, or (c) an unqualified query box search (click on Details to see whether the terms were translated to MeSH).

Some topics *do not* have equivalent MeSH terms. When this occurs, run a free-text or title search on the topic. If the user knows synonyms, these should be included.

If the supplemental title search appears to be too narrow, a free-text search, such as Text Word, which searches titles, abstracts, MeSH, and so on, can be used.

How It Works

The workings of MeSH are described in detail in Chapter 2.

Keep in Mind

Medical librarians are excellent sources of information on MEDLINE search strategies and techniques. When in doubt, contact a medical reference librarian.

Medical Subject Heading (MeSH) Examples

The following examples demonstrate two approaches to MeSH searching. The first uses a title search to "bootstrap" to the MeSH terms; the second uses the MeSH browser.

Example 1: Recent articles on the prevention of community-acquired pneumonia. Locate recent articles on the prevention of community-acquired pneumonia.

Type *prevent* AND "community-acquired pneumonia"* into the query box, but ***do not*** click Go. Instead, click Limits (**A**).

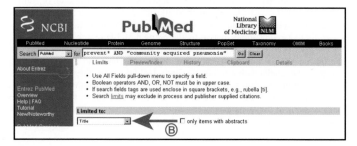

Choose Title (**B**) from the All Fields pull-down menu. Click Go.

Locate a citation or two that seems relevant. *Avoid* the in-process or supplied by publisher records as they do not have MeSH terms. Click on the citation's checkbox (**A**), change the display to Citation (**B**), and click on the Display button (**C**) to show the citation's MeSH terms.

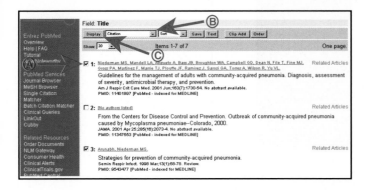

The second citation that was selected, *Strategies for Prevention of Community-Acquired Pneumonia,* contains the MeSH terms shown.

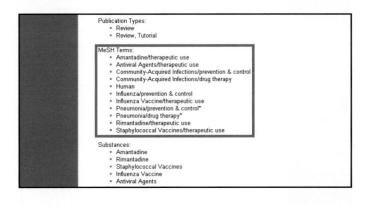

Combining both "Community-Acquired Infections/prevention & control" and "Pneumonia/prevention & control" will result in an *extremely* focused search. To use the MeSH browser to plug these into the search, click on the link to the MeSH browser.

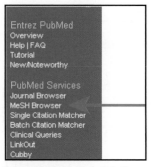

Type *pneumonia* and click Go.

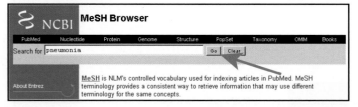

The browser shows where *pneumonia* resides relative to the broader and narrower MeSH terms. To add the subheading "Prevention and Control" to Pneumonia, click on the Detailed Display link.

The Detailed Display provides the searcher with a number of options. The search can be focused using subheadings or Restrict to Major Topic (**A**). Do Not Explode can also be selected if the searcher *does not* want PubMed to retrieve narrower MeSH terms (this option is rarely used by the author). Select the subheading Prevention and Control (**B**) and click the Add button (**C**).

Follow a similar process for community-acquired infections. Type *community-acquired infections* and click Go (**D**).

Click Detailed Display (**E**).

Select Prevention and Control (**A**) and click Add (**B**). (Note that the subject heading Community-Acquired Infections was added in 1994.)

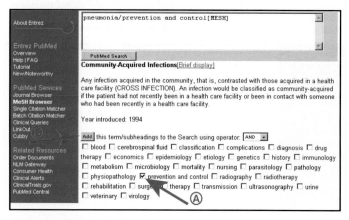

Click the PubMed Search (**C**) button to run the search.

The search retrieved 28 citations. Limit the search to English, 1998 to present. Click the word Limits, not the checkbox (**D**).

NOTE: Although the Title limit is still set, it is ignored. Selecting MeSH terms from the browser added a MeSH field tag to the search statement; this takes precedence over the Title Word search limit.

Select English from the Languages pull-down menu, type *1998* in the From box to the right of Publication Date (**A**). Click Go (**B**).

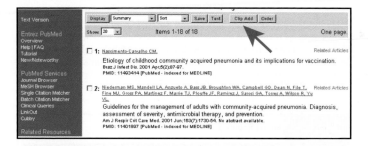

The searcher retrieved 18 citations. Store these temporarily in the Clipboard. Click Clip Add to save all the citations.

At this point, the author usually supplements his MeSH search with another, slightly broader, title or free-text search to retrieve citations that lack MeSH terms (i.e., in-process and supplied by publisher) or those that might have been inconsistently indexed. In this case, a supplemental title search of *(control* OR prevent* OR prophyla*) AND "community-acquired pneumonia"* failed to retrieve anything new or relevant.

Click the Clipboard link (**A**) to retrieve the 18 citations from the earlier search.

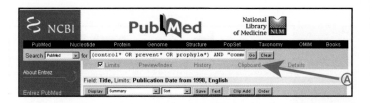

Once the Display is changed to Abstract (**B**) and Pub Date has been chosen as the Sort order (**C**), the user can download, print, or order these 18 citations.

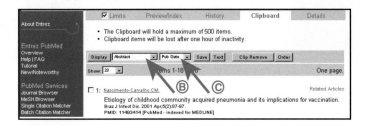

Example 2: Current treatment strategies for Parkinson disease. The goal is to locate some reviews of current treatment strategies for Parkinson disease. The topic is a large one, so the user will want to use MeSH, subheadings, major topic restriction, publication types, and date limits to focus the search. (This example uses the MeSH browser to locate MeSH and subheadings). Click on the link to the MeSH browser, type *Parkinson disease*, and click Go.

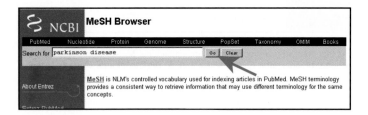

The MeSH browser maps to the MeSH term *Parkinson disease*. Click on the Detailed Display to begin adding subheadings to Parkinson disease.

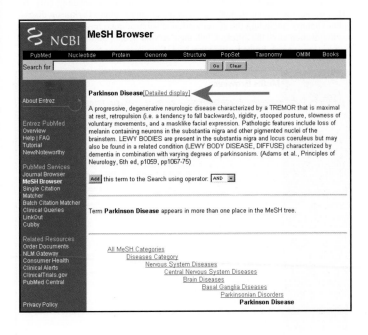

Select Therapy (**A**). In PubMed, this will automatically search *all* treatment or therapy-related subheadings (e.g., Drug Therapy, Diet Therapy, Surgery, Radiotherapy, Nursing, Prevention and Control, Rehabilitation).

To focus the search, select Restrict Search to Major Topic headings only (**B**). This means the search should only retrieve citations where Parkinson disease plus Therapy (including the aforementioned subheadings) have been identified as major themes of the article. Click the PubMed Search button to proceed and apply some search limits by clicking Add (**C**).

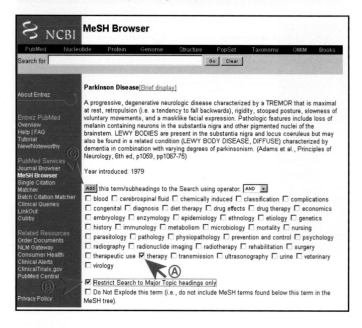

Click Limits (**D**).

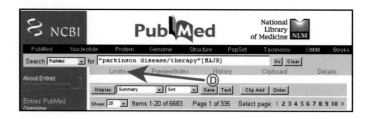

Select publication type as Review, language as English, Human studies, and publication date from 2000 to present (**A**). Click Go (**B**).

Select the citations of particular relevance and then click Clip Add (**C**) to store them in the Clipboard.

To run a supplemental search to retrieve any ultracurrent in-process citations, uncheck the Limits checkbox (**A**) and then click on the word Limits.

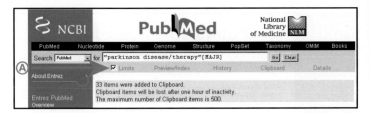

The terms used in the supplemental search (in this case, a title search) are limited only by time and imagination. The following search should retrieve the more obviously relevant citations: *parkinson* AND (manage* OR current OR review OR overview OR guideline*)*.

Select Title from the All Fields pull-down menu. Limit to English language and 2000 to present. Be *sure* to deselect Review and Human, otherwise the unindexed in-process and supplied-by-publisher citations will be lost (**B**). Click Go (**C**).

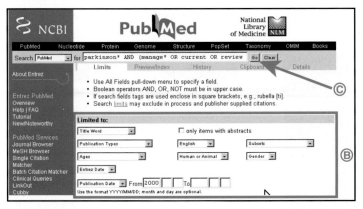

This search identified some new, relevant citations (**D**).

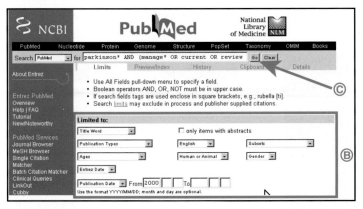

After selecting the relevant citations from the title search, click Clip Add to save them to the Clipboard. Click on Clipboard (**A**) to retrieve the stored citations. Change the Display format to Abstract (**B**), and choose Pub Date as the sort order (**C**). At this point, the user could print, save, or order.

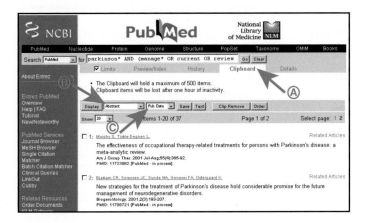

SEARCHING USING FIELD ABBREVIATIONS (TAGS)

On occasion, searching PubMed with search field abbreviations rather than pull-down menus may be faster and more efficient. The abbreviations, or tags, are easy to use, and they can be entered along with the search terms directly into the query box. Tags need to be enclosed in square brackets, and they must *follow* the search term (e.g., *bloor [au] AND angiogenesis [ti]*). Tags are not case sensitive.

To run a field tag search, simply enter the search terms and the PubMed field tags into the query box and click Go.

Some particularly useful field tags are listed below.

Tag	Use and Example
[MH]	MeSH. Useful if one *knows* what the MeSH term is
	otitis media [mh] AND amoxicillin [mh]
	atopic dermatitis/drug therapy [mh] AND ketoconazole [mh]
[MAJR]	MeSH term must be a major topic of the article
	dysentery, bacillary/diagnosis [majr] AND sensitivity and specificity [mh]
[TI]	Title
	shigellosis [ti] AND butler [au]
[PS]	Personal name as subject. Use it to locate articles *about* a particular person
	pauling l [ps]
[TW]	Title Word—this includes title, abstract, MeSH terms, subheadings, and chemical substance names
	spondylolisthesis [tw] AND dysreflexia [tw]
[SH]	Subheading. Often used when a *direct* MeSH/Subheading linkage is not possible
	orphan drug production [mh] AND trends [sh]
[MH:NOEXP]	Do not explode the MeSH term; that is, do not search the MeSH term's narrower MeSH terms
	pneumonia [mh:noexp] AND drug resistance, microbial [mh]
[PT]	Publication type
	shigellosis [ti] AND review [pt]
[LANG]	Language. First three letters of language (some exceptions [e.g., jpn = Japanese])
	shigellosis [ti] AND eng [lang]
[DP]	Publication date. Use the following format: YYYY/MM/DD (month and day are optional); use the colon (:) for a date range
	malaria vaccines [mh] AND 1998:2002 [dp]
	ards [ti] AND 1995 [dp]
	afonso [au] AND 1998/10/06 [dp]

Post-Search Data Management

PRINTING, SAVING, DOWNLOADING, AND E-MAILING

Printing Citations

Printing Everything

When printing citations, the user should ensure that the number listed in Show (the default is 20) is greater than the number he or she intends to print. Why? If 100 citations were found, a display of only 20 citations means that the user will have to print five separate screens of 20 citations per screen. So, in this example of 70 citations, change Show to "100" (**A**) and click the Display button (**B**).

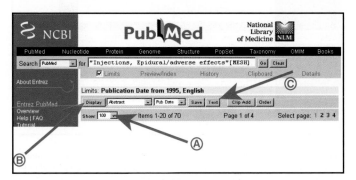

Now all the citations will be listed on one screen, and all the user must do is to click the Web browser's Print button once. The limit for displayed citations per screen is 500; generally, the searcher will not print more than this. Click the Web browser's Print button, and the records will print with the various graphical elements of PubMed (icons, sidebar, etc.).

Text button. A more efficient method for printing uses the Text button. Make the same selections as those listed above, but click the Text button (**C**) before using the Web browser's Print button. Text will display the citations without sidebars, icons, or any other graphics—just the citations, which are listed efficiently without wasted space.

```
1: Am J Phys Med Rehabil 2001 Aug;80(8):618-621

Persistent hiccup associated with thoracic epidural injection.

Slipman CW, Shin CH, Patel RK, Braverman DL, Lenrow DA, Ellen MI, Nematbakhsh
MA.
```

Regardless of which method is chosen, the Web browser's Print button (**A**) can be used to print the citations.

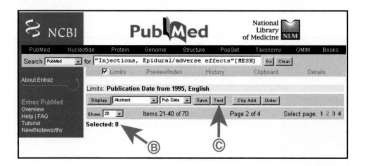

Printing Selected Citations

If the user has been selecting citations with checkboxes but has *not* saved them to the Clipboard, the total will be listed next to the word Selected. In this case, eight records have been selected (**B**).

Again, the searcher must make sure the number listed in Show is a number greater than the number he or she intends to print; he or she can then choose a display format (e.g., Abstract) and a sort order (e.g., Pub Date). The searcher should then click the Display button. Again, the Text button (**C**) can be used to display the records in the most economical format; the Web browser's Print button is then used to print the citations.

Printing from the Clipboard

If the searcher has been using the Clip Add feature to save citations and he or she is ready to print, he or she can click on Clipboard (**A**). Note the number of citations saved (**B**), change the number listed in Show to a number greater than the number to be printed, choose a Display format (e.g., Abstract) and a Sort option (e.g., by publication date), and then click the Text button (**C**). Click the browser's Print button to print the clipboard's citations.

Saving or Downloading Citations

Citations from PubMed can be saved (downloaded) as a simple text file to a floppy or hard disc and then imported, e-mailed, or archived.

NOTE: If one is planning to import the citations into a citation management program like EndNote, downloading the citations in the MEDLINE format is *critical* (see "Using Citation Management Software").

Downloading Everything

To download *all* citations from a particular search without selecting individual citations, choose a display format (e.g., Abstract) and, if desired, a sort order (e.g., publication date). Click on the Save button (**D**). Name the file and add the extension ".txt" (e.g., mysearch.txt) (**E**). Decide where to save the file; one option would be a folder, with a name such as "PubMed Searches".

Downloading Selected Citations

If the user has been selecting citations with checkboxes and *not* saving them to the Clipboard, he or she will see the total number of citations selected in the area below the Show pull-down menu (**A**). Choose a Display format (e.g., Abstract) and, if desired, a sort order (e.g., Publication Date). Click on the Save button (**B**). Name the file and add the extension ".txt" (e.g., mysearch.txt) (**C**). As mentioned above, decide where to save the file.

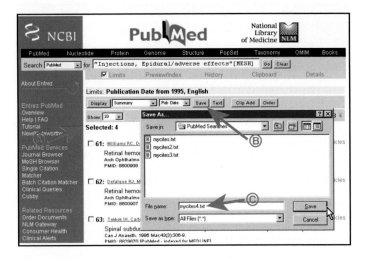

Downloading from the Clipboard

If one has been using the Clipboard and is ready to download, click on the word Clipboard. Once in the Clipboard, the user follows the same instructions as listed in the preceding section (i.e., choose a Display format and so on).

E-mailing Citations

Quick Overview

PubMed currently lacks an e-mail option *per se*; however, *if* the Web browser is configured for e-mail, one can download the citations and can then send them as an e-mail attachment.

Example: E-mailing a set of citations. To e-mail a set of citations from PubMed, first set the Display and sort options as desired (see "Saving or Downloading Citations"). After clicking the Save button, give the file a name and a ".txt" extension (**A**).

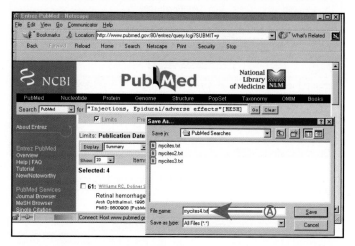

After saving the citations, pull up an e-mail message template (Netscape version 4.5 is used here) (**B**).

After typing in the e-mail address, go to the "Attach" pull-down menu and choose "File."

Locate the citations that were downloaded, select the file, and click the Open button.

Click Send. The file has now been sent.

STORING SEARCHES USING THE CUBBY

Quick Overview

One of the more attractive features of PubMed is its stored search utility, which is called the *Cubby*. Searchers can run searches and download citations and can then store the search strategy. Searchers can log in to Cubby at a later date, re-run their stored searches, and retrieve *new* citations added to PubMed since the last search.

Other systems (Ovid is a prime example) extend this feature one step further by automating the update function. As new citations are added, they are compared with stored searches and the results are automatically e-mailed to the searcher. The individual does not need to log in and rerun the search; it is done automatically. PubMed, although it does not have this feature, can store up to 100 searches per user name.

Example

An individual has an interest in Whipple disease. He or she runs a comprehensive search on Whipple disease and downloads citations, perhaps importing them into a citation manager, such as EndNote. At this point, the user feels up-to-date with the journal literature on the topic. To stay up-to-date, he or she could save the search strategy in the Cubby. To do so, the user clicks on the link to the Cubby.

The user should register with Cubby or log in (if he or she already has a Cubby user name and password).

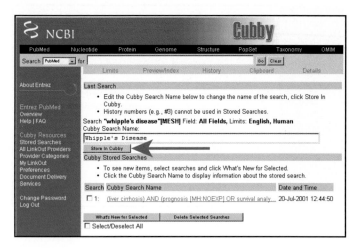

Once the user has logged in, the Cubby Stored Search page will appear. If the user saved other searches, they will be listed toward the bottom of the page.

Cubby assumes the user wants to save the last search and uses those search terms as the default Cubby Search Name. In the example shown, the default Search Name was changed to *Whipple's disease*. Click the Store in Cubby button to save the search.

Later (e.g., a couple of months), one could connect to PubMed, log in to Cubby, select the saved search (**A**), and then click on the What's New for Selected button (**B**).

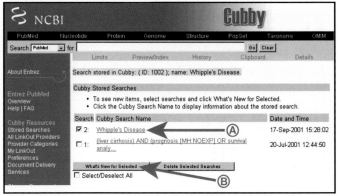

Only new citations that have been added to PubMed since the last search will be retrieved.

USING CITATION MANAGEMENT SOFTWARE

Quick Overview

Citation management software programs, also known as reprint or bibliographic management software, are terrific tools that can help users organize file cabinets full of article reprints or megabytes worth of downloaded PubMed citations. Even more amazing than this is the ability of these programs to format manuscript bibliographies quickly and easily. Simply select a bibliography style (e.g., *Annals of Internal Medicine, JAMA: The Journal of the American Medical Association, Science,* or *Journal of Biological Chemistry*), click a button, and the in-text citations of the manuscript are instantly converted into a nicely formatted bibliography.

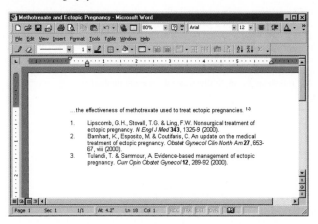

Below is a screen shot of an EndNote (version 5) Library of 22 imported PubMed citations. One of the citations has been opened.

Although a detailed description of these programs is beyond the scope of this handbook, the next page illustrates techniques for importing citations into EndNote.

Importing

PubMed citations can be imported into a citation management program such as EndNote in the following two ways: (a) searching PubMed from within End-Note (the downside of this approach is that the PubMed search interface is *significantly* more powerful than that which is provided by EndNote) or (b) downloading the PubMed citations in the MEDLINE format and importing them using EndNote's Import option.

The following example illustrates the second method.

Step 1

When downloading citations from PubMed, be sure to choose the MEDLINE display format (**A**). The field tags that are part of this format help integrate the information from the citation into the citation management database.

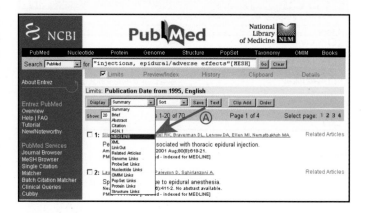

Step 2

Be sure to save the citations with a ".txt" extension after the filename (**B**). This ensures that the file is saved in a simple, easy-to-read format that will not confuse the citation manager.

Step 3

Next, be sure to indicate the source (e.g., PubMed) of the downloaded citations. Do this within the citation manager (in EndNote, use Import Filters).

Step 4

Import the saved PubMed records with the EndNote Import option. Find the file with the Choose File button. Select an Import Option—in this case, PubMed (NLM). Choose Discard Duplicates to delete duplicate records. Click the Import button.

Mission accomplished! The result is 71 records successfully imported into the user's EndNote library. The user can now select and insert the records into a manuscript and can then use EndNote to generate a bibliography from the in-text citations.

ORDERING ARTICLES THROUGH LOANSOME DOC

Quick Overview

PubMed provides access to several document delivery services, including NLM's venerable Loansome Doc. To use Loansome Doc, one must first establish an agreement with a participating medical library. Fees for the service vary.

If one is affiliated with an institution that has a medical library, that library should be contacted first for more information. Otherwise, contact the Regional Medical Library by telephone at 1-800-338-RMLS (7657), Monday through Friday, from 8:30 AM to 5:00 PM in all time zones, to locate the nearest medical library.

Other commercial document delivery services are also available. To link to one of these services, log in to Cubby (see "Storing Searches Using the Cubby" for more details) and select the Document Delivery Services link on the left sidebar.

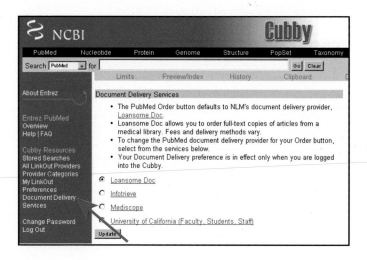

Keep in mind that rates for these services vary. The University of California (UC) link shown in this example is, of course, for UC faculty, staff, and students.

Select desired citations and click on the Order button.

Type in a user ID and password and then click Go.

REFERENCES

1. Clinical Alerts home page. Available at: http://www.nlm.nih.gov/databases/alerts/clinical_alerts.html. Accessed May 2002.
2. MEDLARS Management Section, United States National Library of Medicine. *Keeping up with NLM's PubMed®, the NLM Gateway and ClinicalTrials.gov*. Bethesda, MD: National Library of Medicine, 2001.

CHAPTER 4
Ovid MEDLINE

Overview, Screens, and Tools

Ovid Technologies evolved from the amalgamation of two database vendors—CD-PLUS, which had developed a highly effective search interface for its collection of CD-ROM–based databases, and BRS Online, an online database vendor with a rich collection of databases in the area of health and medicine.

Like the company itself, the Ovid Web gateway is a bit of a hybrid. BRS Online command-line search syntax is still available for "power searchers," and aspects of the old CD-PLUS searching interface are still evident in the current Web gateway interface

The interface, one of the most intuitive Web-based MEDLINE search interfaces available, plays a large role in Ovid's popularity. A stated goal of the company is to develop software that "takes advantage of the content and unique features of individual databases, combining content and technology" (1). Nowhere is this more apparent than in its Web interface to MEDLINE. Powerful mapping algorithms smoothly integrate Medical Subject Headings (MeSH) and subheadings into the search process in ways that are both intuitive and empowering to the novice searcher. Although many search systems (e.g., PubMed) provide access to the same MEDLINE features (MeSH, subheadings, etc.), they often do so in a less clear-cut, less well-integrated way.

NOTE: Local configuration decisions have a significant impact on the appearance and functionality of Ovid databases such as MEDLINE. The examples in this chapter may show some screens or features that are not available at a particular institution.

OVERVIEW

Databases

Ovid offers more than 90 databases collectively known as *Databases@Ovid*, many of which are in the areas of the health and life sciences. Ovid packs a number of value-added features into these databases, the exact configuration of which depends on how Ovid is implemented at a specific institution. The following features are particularly noteworthy:

- **AutoAlerts.** Regularly and automatically runs saved searches and e-mails the results
- **OpenLinks.** Links to non-Ovid external full text
- Automatic mapping of search terms to a database's subject headings
- Multifile searching with duplicate deletion

Other Products and Services

In addition to its databases, Ovid offers a wide range of products and services, many of which are clinically oriented.

Online Books

Books@Ovid is a collection of more than 50 medical, nursing, and pharmacology textbooks.

Online Journals

Journals@Ovid is a database of more than 530 fully indexed, full-text electronic journals, a growing percentage of which are being rendered in portable document format (PDF). The full-text articles are searchable, and they are linked to Ovid's database citations. *Access* to the full-text, however, depends on the specific institution's journal subscription profile.

OpenLinks is a supplement to Ovid's Journals@Ovid collection. It links citations to non-Ovid full-text providers.

Decision Support

MedWeaver is a decision support tool that generates a differential diagnosis based on a set of user-submitted symptoms and patient characteristics. The tool includes a disease look-up module and an integrated Ovid MEDLINE search option.

Clineguide is another decision support tool available from Ovid. Clineguide provides recommendations for the clinical management and treatment of a particular condition. The following three navigation pathways guide the user through the system: Disease, Drug Choice, and Quick Drug.

Education

MedCases is a problem-based learning tool designed primarily for medical students and residents. Using simulated or virtual patients, users can generate differential diagnoses, order laboratory tests, search Ovid online resources, consult additional information about the patient's history, determine treatment, determine the final diagnosis, and so on.

Evidence-Based Medicine

Ovid's evidence-based medicine (EBM) resources include EBM Reviews (EBMR) and Clinical Evidence (produced by the publisher of the *British Medical Journal* [*BMJ*]). The EBMR currently contains four separate resources as follows: the American College of Physicians (ACP) Journal Club, the Cochrane Controlled Trials Register, the Cochrane Database of Systematic Reviews, and the Database of Abstracts of Reviews of Effectiveness (DARE). These are described in more detail in Appendix 1. Clinical Evidence is a resource that summarizes the latest evidence for the effectiveness of common treatments, as well as prevention strategies for various conditions.

Personal Digital Assistants

Ovid@Hand is a relatively new application developed for personal digital assistants (PDAs). The tool provides information about drugs and drug interactions, stores tables of contents for various journals, and allows users to submit stored searches to Ovid databases.

Customizing Ovid

How Ovid looks and operates depends on the method of access that is being used (i.e., via the Ovid Web Gateway or via a CD-ROM on a stand-alone workstation), what features have been configured at a particular location, and the subscribed resources.

Lane Medical Library, at the Stanford University Medical Center, for example, accesses Ovid via its Web Gateway and subscribes to more than a half dozen databases and to several of Ovid's subject-based journal collections. Activating some search features (e.g., automatic MeSH explosion) are decisions that were made locally by Lane Library.

Getting Started

Before beginning to search, connect to Ovid Online. Remember that, unlike PubMed, Ovid requires a subscription.

The method that is used to connect depends on how Ovid has been configured. Off-site users may have to log in using the following screen:

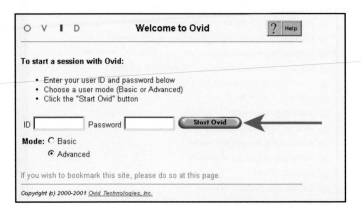

When searching on-site at a subscribing institution, the user generally will be seen as a legitimate user (via the user's computer's Internet Protocol [IP] address); he or she will thus be able to bypass a log-in and will simply click Start Ovid. Alternatively, a link on the institution's home page may take the user to the Ovid database selection window or directly into a particular Ovid database.

Some special features (e.g., AutoAlerts) may be accessible only by logging in with a particular identification (ID) and password (these are often distributed through the institution's library). Also, pay-as-you-go subscribers may need to enter user IDs and passwords.

Some institutions provide proxy off-site access to Ovid. In these instances, when a user accesses the Web via a commercial Internet service provider, he or she might be blocked because Ovid has no way to know the affiliation of the user. The institution, however, can set up a proxy link that can verify the user's legitimacy via a locally issued password and user name.

Choose a Database

After log-in, the user probably will see a list of databases to which the institution has subscribed. The user can select either one or, if multifile searching has been enabled, up to five databases. After selecting a database (or databases), the main Ovid search screen will appear.

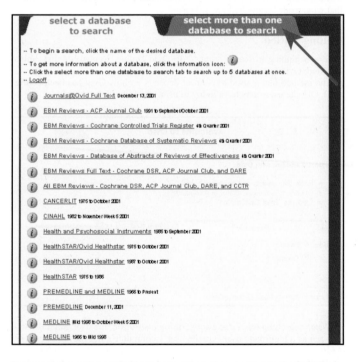

For more information on Ovid products and services, connect to the Ovid Technologies website at http://www.ovid.com.

ADVANTAGES AND DISADVANTAGES OF OVID MEDLINE

Advantages

- A highly intuitive interface that promotes the use of MEDLINE's value-added indexing information (e.g., MeSH, subheadings); excellent MeSH tools.
- Excellent phrase, adjacency, and frequency searching.
- Links to many full-text journals.
- Search History screen prominently displayed.
- AutoAlert search feature.
- Easy-to-use save, display, e-mail, and print options.
- Multifile search capability, including duplicate deletion.

Disadvantages

- Web connection sometimes slow but is improving.
- Not free; subscription is required.
- Only a small percentage of Journals@Ovid articles in PDF (changing).
- Lacks some of the fancy search features offered by PubMed (e.g., Clinical Query, Related Article).

ADVANCED SEARCH SCREEN

Ⓐ
O V I D **MEDLINE**
<1966 to October Week 1 2001> ? Help

Author Title Journal Search Fields Tools Combine Limit Basic Change Database Logoff

Ⓑ

#	Search History	Results	Display
1	exp Pregnancy, Ectopic/	7696	Display
2	exp METHOTREXATE/	20987	Display
3	1 and 2	516	Display
4	limit 3 to (human and english language and yr=1990-2001)	369	Display

⦿ Saved Searches   ⦿ Save Search History   ⦿ Delete Searches

Ⓒ
Enter **Keyword** or phrase: ☑ Map Term to Subject Heading

[   ] **Perform Search**

Ⓓ
Limit to:
☐ Ovid Full Text Available ☐ Human ☐ English Language ☐ Review Articles ☐ Abstracts
☐ EBM Reviews ☐ Latest Update
Publication Year [· ▾]-[· ▾]

Ask A Librarian

Search Screens

Ovid offers searchers two primary search screens—Basic and Advanced. The Advanced screen is so well designed and easy to use that most searchers ignore the *extremely* simple Basic screen.

Search Icons (A)

Author. Search for an author (not recommended for most author searches; see "Author Searching").

Title. Search for words in titles.

Journal. Search for citations from a particular journal.

Search Fields. Search any field within a database record (e.g., page number, volume number, publication year).

Tools. This feature, used primarily by professional searchers, provides navigational aids to MeSH. Tree displays a graphical representation of a MeSH term relative to broader and narrower MeSH terms. Permuted Index displays MeSH terms that contain a particular word (e.g., MeSH terms containing the word *pulmonary*). Scope Note provides searchers with additional information about a MeSH term, sometimes even a definition of the MeSH term itself. Explode automatically searches for a MeSH term and its narrower MeSH terms (e.g., exploding *migraine* retrieves *classic migraine* and *common migraine*). Subheading retrieves the subheadings that apply to a particular MeSH term (e.g., pregnancy, ectopic/diagnosis).

Combine. This tool enables the combination of search sets with the Boolean operators *AND* and *OR*.

Limit. This feature restricts the search using a remarkable collection of limits (e.g., age groups, languages, gender).

Basic. Clicking on this icon displays Ovid's basic search interface.

Change Database. This switches the searcher to another database and provides an option for automatically rerunning the search in the new database.

Log-off. This button is used to end the search session and disconnect from Ovid.

Search History (B)

The Search History window displays the search number, search syntax, retrieved citations, and the display button.

Saved Searches. This option enables the user to retrieve or delete any saved searches.

Save Search History. A user can save a search, temporarily, permanently, or as an AutoAlert (see "Saving Searches" in "Postsearch Data Management").

Delete Searches. This button is used to delete any or all of the current search sets.

Command Line (C)

Command Line. Search terms and search commands can be entered on this line.

Map Term to Subject Heading. If this option is selected, Ovid will attempt to match search terms to a MeSH term.

Limit To

This is a short list of some of the more common search limits. Search options vary depending on the database (see "Limiting Searches").

Ask a Librarian. This customizable search limit allows searchers to submit questions, along with their search strategies, electronically to a librarian or another information professional.

BASIC SEARCH SCREEN

Search Icons (A)

Advanced links to the Advanced search screen.

Change Database switches to another database.

Log-off ends the search session and disconnects from Ovid.

Command Lines (B)

Keywords Command Line enables a broad search of titles, abstracts, registry number words, and MeSH.

Author Command Line gives the user the ability to search by author.

Limits (C)

Limit to supplies the same basic limits as those available on the advanced search page.

Ask a Librarian is customizable. It allows searchers to submit questions, along with their search strategies, electronically to a librarian or another information professional.

DISPLAYING CITATIONS

Display Button. To display citations, simply click the Display button in the Search History box or just scroll down the page.

Citation Title Display

Navigation Buttons (A). Clicking on the Display button takes the user to a new page with navigational buttons at the top. The middle button returns the searcher to the Ovid MEDLINE main search page. The other two take the user either back or forward one citation.

Results, Citations Displayed, and so on (B). "Results of your search" shows the search strategy. "Citations displayed" shows which citations are being displayed and provides a button that allows jumping to a particular citation. Customize Display allows the user to change how citations are displayed (see "Customizing the Display"). The user can set which fields are displayed, can adjust the citation format, can change how many citations are displayed per page, and can even alter how search terms are highlighted.

Citation Manager, Help, and Log-off (C). Use the Citation Manager to prepare citations for downloading, printing, or e-mailing (see "Citation Manager" in "Postsearch Data Management").

OpenLinks. This is available for purchase from Ovid Technologies.

> ☐ 27. Jacobs JE. Birnbaum BA. Macari M. Megibow AJ. Israel G. Maki DD. Aguiar AM. Langlotz CP. Acute **appendicitis**: comparison of helical CT diagnosis focused technique with oral contrast material versus nonfocused technique with oral and intravenous contrast material. **[Journal Article]** *Radiology.* *220(3):683-90, 2001 Sep.* Held by Ovid Technologies
> **UI**: 21417816
>
> Abstract • Complete Reference • OpenLink Full Text (HTML) • OpenLink Full Text (PDF) • Journal Website

OpenLinks supplements the full-text available through Journals@Ovid by linking to non-Ovid electronic journals and external content providers. Depending on a variety of factors (e.g., the local configuration of Ovid, the configuration of external provider's websites, and the electronic availability of full-text formats), the following links may be seen: OvidLink Full Text (HTML), OvidLink Full Text (PDF), and Journal Website.

Abstract, Complete Reference, and Ovid Full Text. Abstract shows the basic citation with the abstract. Complete Reference shows the MEDLINE citation with the abstract and MeSH terms. Ovid Full Text, which requires a subscription to an Ovid full-text collection, links to the full-text version of a particular document.

> ☐ 1. Shapira MY. Muszkat M. Braunstein I. Gotsman I. Co-occurrence of **hepato**cellular carcinoma and lymphoma in patients with hepatitis C virus cirrhosis. **[Journal Article]** *Journal of Clinical Gastroenterology. 32(4):368-9, 2001 Apr.* Held by Ovid Technologies
> **UI**: 21172951
>
> Abstract • Complete Reference • **Ovid Full Text**

Complete Reference is a particularly important display format because it allows viewing of MeSH terms; these can then be used to find other similar citations.

> **Title**
>   Co-occurrence of **hepato**cellular carcinoma and lymphoma in patients with hepatitis C virus cirrhosis.
> **Source**
>   Journal of Clinical Gastroenterology. 32(4):368-9, 2001 Apr.
> **NLM Journal Code**
>   ibg, 7910017
> **Journal Subset**
>   Index Medicus
> **Country of Publication**
>   United States
> **MeSH Subject Headings**
>   Aged
>   *Carcinoma, **Hepato**cellular / vi [Virology]
>   Case Report
>   *Hepatitis C / co [Complications]
>   Human
>   *Liver Neoplasms / vi [Virology]
>   *Lymphoma / vi [Virology]
>   Male
>   *Neoplasms, Multiple Primary
>   *Stomach Neoplasms / vi [Virology]
>   Venous Thrombosis / co [Complications]
> **Abstract**
>   The association of hepatitis C virus (HCV) with neoplasia is not completely understood. Hepatitis C virus is

Customizing the Display

To change how the lists of citations are displayed either permanently or semipermanently, click Customize Display.

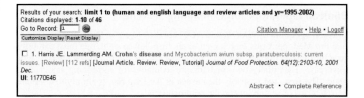

Select For this Session (**A**) so the display will revert to the default title display following the log-out. Then choose a display, such as abstracts and MeSH terms (**B**), and a format (**C**). Changing how many citations are displayed per page is also possible (**D**).

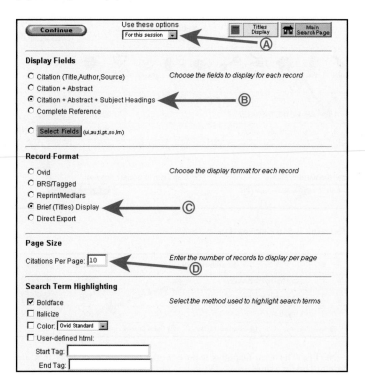

BASIC TOOLS

Ovid offers the searcher a potent set of search tools, several of which are more powerful than their PubMed counterparts.

Boolean Operators and Combining Searches

Boolean operators (*AND*, *OR*, and *NOT*) are easy to use in Ovid. Because Ovid, like PubMed, performs search operations from left to right, one must carefully structure search queries. Boolean operators can be used in either uppercase or lowercase. Essentially two methods are available for combining searches in Ovid. The first, and probably the easiest in the long run, is simply to combine search terms or search sets on the command line.

Example: Combining Search Sets

To combine the two search sets below (**A**), simply type *1 and 2* (**B**), and click the Perform Search button (**C**).

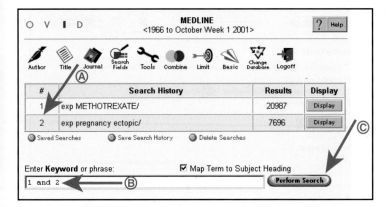

The result is 516 citations (**D**).

#	Search History	Results	Display
1	exp METHOTREXATE/	20987	Display
2	exp pregnancy ectopic/	7696	Display
3	1 and 2	516	Display

Saved Searches   Save Search History   Delete Searches

NOTE: The term-mapping feature works best with concepts that are searched one at a time.

Example: Inadvertent Deactivation of Term Mapping

Locate citations on *vitamin c and kidney stones*.

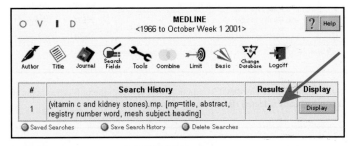

The terms failed to map to subject headings. Instead, the field tag ".mp" means that Ovid ran a free-text search (Titles, Abstracts, and Subject Headings) of the terms *vitamin C* and *kidney stones*.

#	Search History	Results	Display
1	(vitamin c and kidney stones).mp. [mp=title, abstract, registry number word, mesh subject heading]	4	Display

Therefore, as one of Ovid's best features is its ability to map to MeSH terms, search each topic separately and then combine the resulting search sets to take advantage of this.

Example: Combining Sets on the Command Line

Locate articles by *NE Shumway* that discuss either *coronary artery bypass* or *heart transplantation*. Combine the sets (**A**) on the command line (**B**).

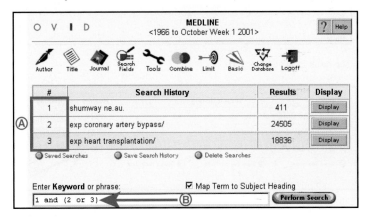

#	Search History	Results	Display
1	shumway ne.au.	411	Display
2	exp coronary artery bypass/	24505	Display
3	exp heart transplantation/	18836	Display

The second method for combining searches takes advantage of the Combine icon; this method is a bit more cumbersome.

Example: Using the Combine Icon

To combine search sets 1 and 2, click the Combine icon (**A**).

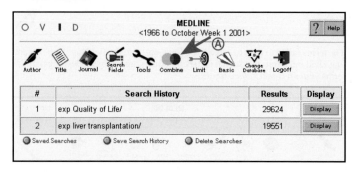

Next, select search sets 1 and 2 and click on *AND* from the pull-down menu if it is not already selected (**B**). Click the Continue button (**C**).

The result is 248 citations (**D**).

Truncation and Wild Cards

Ovid provides an impressive array of truncation and wild card options. What follows are brief summaries of some of the more popular options:

Unlimited Truncation. Use the dollar sign ($) to retrieve terms that begin with a particular character string. For example, a title search on *allerg$* will retrieve citations with terms beginning with the letters *allerg* (e.g., allergy, allergic, allergies).

Note that *allergy* appears in the title of one citation (**A**) and *allergens* in another (**B**).

If unlimited truncation retrieves too many citations, the user can limit the number of characters that follow the search term. For example, *allerg$2* will retrieve *allergic* but not *allergies*.

Truncation is also a handy tool for the spelling-impaired user. For instance, what is the correct spelling of *cytomegalovirus*? The user can run a title search on the term using truncation at the point at which he or she is unsure of the spelling (e.g., *cytomeg$*) and can then look to see how the term is spelled.

Wild Cards. In Ovid, the question mark (?) can be used as a wild card to represent one or zero characters. The wild card, unlike the unlimited truncation symbol, can be used *inside* the search term.

Example: Locate Citations with Alternate Spellings of a Term

To locate citations that mention either *armor* or *armour*, run a search on *armo?r*.

For some searches, the user might wish to combine both wild cards *and* truncation. For example, to locate citations that mention *color* or *colour* and *analog* or *analogue*, type *colo?r and analog$*.

Enter **Keyword** or phrase: ☑ Map Term to Subject Heading

`colo?r and analog$`   **Perform Search**

Remember that one of Ovid's greatest advantages over PubMed is its ability to truncate without restriction—PubMed is limited to the first 150 variations, whereas Ovid gets them all.

Nesting with Parentheses

Parentheses force Ovid to perform the operations within the parentheses before moving to operators outside the parentheses. Operations within the deepest set of parentheses are processed first.

Example: Grouping Synonyms

A popular use of parentheses is grouping synonyms. If the user is trying to locate an article on urography for kidney trauma but cannot remember the exact title, he or she could try a title search of *urography AND (trauma$ OR injur$) AND (kidney OR renal)*.

Enter a word or phrase to be searched in the **title**:

`urography AND (trauma$ OR injur$) AND (kidney OR r`   **Perform Search**

Adjacency Searching

The ability to search for terms within a defined proximity of other terms is a powerful tool, one that is well supported by the Ovid system.

Phrase Searching is the the most common type of adjacency searching (e.g., *mad cow disease*). Ovid assumes adjacency for words that are separated by a space.

Example: Phrase Search

A user is trying to locate a citation that mentions the phrase *neurology of Whipple disease* in either the title or abstract. Turn *off* Map Term to Subject Heading so that Ovid will not try to map to a MeSH term. Type in the phrase and then click Perform Search.

```
Enter Keyword or phrase:          □ Map Term to Subject Heading
neurology of whipple's disease          Perform Search
```

NOTE: If the search phrase includes a Boolean operator (*AND*, *OR*, *NOT*), enclose the phrase in quotes (e.g., *"sensitivity and specificity"*). If the phrase is not enclosed in quotes, Ovid will run searches of the word, and the term *sensitivity* and the term *specificity* in any order, not just for occurrences of the two terms next to one another.

In this example, Ovid performed a free-text search (the field tag ".mp." indicates a search of titles, abstracts, and so on) of the phrase *neurology of Whipple's disease*.

```
Results of your search: neurology of whipple's disease.mp. [mp=title, abstract, registry
number word, mesh subject heading]
Citation displayed: 1 of 1
Go to Record: 1  Go               Citation Manager • Help • Logoff
Customize Display  Reset Display

□ 1. Anderson M. Neurology of Whipple's disease. [Editorial] Journal of Neurology,
Neurosurgery & Psychiatry. 68(1):2-5, 2000 Jan.
UI: 20069959
                              Complete Reference • Ovid Full Text
```

Adjacency

Ovid's adjacency operator, ADJ, can be used with a numeric value to designate the distance between search terms and phrases. For example, *vitamin c adj4 common cold* retrieves citations where *vitamin C* is within four words of *common cold*, whether four words ahead or four words behind.

```
Enter Keyword or phrase:          □ Map Term to Subject Heading
vitamin c adj4 common cold          Perform Search
```

Frequency

Another interesting tool offered by Ovid is Frequency, which can be used to retrieve citations containing a word or phrase occurring *X* number of times. The idea is that, if the search terms are mentioned frequently, then the chances that the citation is relevant to the search are greater. Ovid allows frequency searching of only one field at a time (e.g., Abstract), so a multifield search (e.g., title, abstract, and MeSH) cannot be used. The format for a Frequency query is as follows:

Search term<period>search field<period><slash>freq
<equals sign>number of times search term must occur

Example: Frequency Searching of an Abstract

Locate citations where otitis media occurs at least five times in an abstract (*oti-*

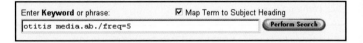

tis media.ab./freq=5).

If the user forgets to put the second period after the field tag, Ovid will automatically add it (see "Command-line Search Syntax and Field Tags").

Command-Line Search Syntax and Field Tags

Before the advent of icons, pull-down menus, and other features of graphical search interfaces, searchers of databases like MEDLINE built their searches using an arcane text-based command syntax. Ovid's graphical Web-based interface does not require searchers to use these exotic commands, but it does allow searchers to use them if they so choose (note that searches in the Search History box are displayed in command-line syntax format). The chief advantage to using command-line search syntax is speed (e.g., typing *smith jm.au* is faster than using Ovid's Author search icon, although the icon does have its uses [see "Author Searching"]).

In the author's experience, the following six field tags (and one command— Explode) are particularly useful:

Author	.au.	*bloor cm.au.*
Title	.ti.	*atopic dermatitis.ti.*
Multipurpose	.mp.	*lung tranplantation.mp.* The fields searched with ".mp." vary depending on the database. In Ovid MEDLINE, .mp. searches titles, abstracts, MeSH terms, and Registry Number Words (see "Glossary" for more info).
Journal	.jn.	*journal of clinical investigation.jn.*
Page	.pg.	*"3".pg.*
Year	.yr.	*"1999".yr.*
Explode	exp	*exp inflammatory bowel diseases* Explode simultaneously searches a MeSH term and its narrower MeSH terms.

NOTE: If the second period after the field tag is omitted, Ovid's error correction will add it automatically.

Example: Locating Citations by Author and Title Terms

To locate citations by N. E. Shumway that mention heart transplantation in the title, type *shumway ne.au and heart transplantation.ti* and then click Perform Search.

Enter **Keyword** or phrase: ☑ Map Term to Subject Heading

shumway ne.au and heart transplantation.ti (Perform Search)

NOTE: When searching numeric fields, like page number or volume number, be sure to place the number in quotes. For example, when searching for citations starting with page number 3, type *"3".pg* . Otherwise, Ovid will think the user wants to rerun the third search (e.g. a search for hepatitis C) in the page number field.

LIMITING SEARCHES

Quick Limits

Most searchers apply restrictions or limits to the searches they run in MED-LINE. One of Ovid's more impressive features is its gigantic collection of search limits. These limits allow the discriminating searcher a great deal of control over the parameters of an Ovid MEDLINE search.

Looking at the preselected search limits located below the command-line search box on the Advanced Search interface is a good starting place (some of the following descriptions were taken from Ovid MEDLINE help screens).

Ovid Full-Text Available. This feature sets limits to the full text; it appears only if the institution has a subscription to the title through Ovid.

Human. This option restricts the search to articles about human subjects; it does include articles that discuss both humans and animals

English Language. This limits the search results to articles written in English.

Review Articles. This is used to specify the "review" article publication type.

Abstracts. Selecting this retrieves only citations with abstracts.

EBM Reviews. The feature restricts the search to studies that have been included by the Cochrane Collaboration when creating a Topic Review or to articles that have been reviewed in the ACP Journal Club, *BMJ* EBM publications, or DARE; it appears only if the institution subscribes to EBM Reviews.

Latest Update. This limit allows searches of recently added citations.

Publication Year. Enter publication date range. Unlike PubMed, one must enter both years (e.g., 1990–2001).

Limits Page

If the user needs more limits than those available on the Advanced Search screen, he or she can simply click the Limit icon, and the following Limits screen will appear:

(A)

Select	#	Search History	Results
○	1	exp pneumococcal pneumonia/dt	491
○	2	exp drug resistance, microbial/	60619
◉	3	1 and 2	142

(B)

Limit to:

- *i* ☐ Human
- *i* ☐ Abstracts
- *i* ☐ Animal
- *i* ☐ AIM Journals
- *i* ☐ Topic Reviews <Cochrane>
- *i* ☐ English Language
- *i* ☐ Ovid Full Text Available
- *i* ☐ Male
- *i* ☐ Evidence Based Medicine Reviews
- *i* ☐ Article Reviews <Best Evidence>
- *i* ☐ Review Articles
- *i* ☐ Latest Update
- *i* ☐ Female
- *i* ☐ All EBMR Article Reviews
- *i* ☐ Article Reviews <DARE>

i Publication Year ☐ - ☐

(C)

To select or remove multiple items from a list below, hold down the Shift, Ctrl, or "Apple" key while selecting.

i Languages

```
·
Afrikaans
Albanian
Arabic
Armenian
Azerbaijani
```

i Age Groups

```
·
All Infant <birth to 23 months>
All Child <0 to 18 years>
All Adult <19 plus years>
Newborn Infant <birth to 1 month>
Infant <1 to 23 months>
```

i Publication Types

```
·
Addresses
Bibliography
Biography
Classical Article
Clinical Conference
```

i Animal Types

```
·
Cats
Cattle
Chick Embryo
Dogs
Goats
```

i Journal Subsets

```
·
AIDS/HIV Journals
AIM Journals
Biotechnology Journals
Communication Journals
Consumer Health Journals
```

Search History (A)

One of the major advantages to the Limits page is the ability to add or reapply search limits to earlier searches. Simply choose the search set, add the search limits, and then click on the Limit Search button.

Single Limit Options (B)

Several of the following descriptions are based on Ovid MEDLINE help screens.

Human, Animal	Restricts the search to either human or animal studies
Abstracts	Restricts the search to citations with abstracts
Abridged Index Medicus (AIM) Journals	Identical to PubMed's Core Clinical Journals; 120 journals that form the core of many small hospital library journal collections
Topic Reviews (Cochrane)	Restricts retrieval to those articles and studies that were included in the creation of a Cochrane review on a topic
English Language	Restricts to English-language articles
Ovid Full Text Available	Provides full text of the article. A growing number of articles are available in PDF
Male, Female	Limits to a particular gender
EBM Reviews	Restricts retrieval to articles or studies that have been included by the Cochrane Collaboration when creating a Topic Review or to articles that have been reviewed in the ACP Journal Club, *BMJ* EBM publications, or DARE (if the institution subscribes to this feature)
Article Reviews (ACP Journal Club)	Restricts retrieval to those articles for which a review exists in the ACP Journal Club database
Article Reviews (DARE)	Restricts retrieval to articles for which a review exists in the DARE database
Review Articles	Limits to review articles
Latest Update	Restricts to the most recent batch of new MEDLINE citations
All EBMR Articles	Restricts retrieval to those articles for which a review exists in either the ACP Journal Club or the DARE databases
Publication Year	Date of publication

Pull-Down Menu Limit Options (C)

Languages	Everything from Afrikaans to Welsh
Age Groups	Infant, newborn to aged, and 80 plus. Ovid also allows the user to choose groupings (e.g., All Child, All Adult). Select more than one age group with the CTRL key for the personal computer (PC) or the Apple key for Macintosh (Macs)

Publication Types	Different types of publications (e.g., review, randomized controlled trial)
Animal Types	Different animals (e.g., cats, dogs, horses)

Journal Subsets: Groups of topically related journals. New subsets may be added as the National Library of Medicine's (NLM's) specialty databases are closed and their journal citations are integrated into MEDLINE (e.g., BIOETHICSLINE, HISTLINE, POPLINE, SPACELINE, and AIDSLINE). The following list gives some of the most popular:

- **Acquired Immunodeficiency Syndrome/Human Immunodeficiency Virus (AIDS/HIV) Journals.** Limits to AIDS/HIV journals.
- **AIM Journals.** Includes 120 core clinical journals. AIM, an abridged version of the *Index Medicus* print index, is synonymous with PubMed's Core Clinical Journals subset.
- **Dentistry Journals.** Limits to dentistry journals.
- **Consumer Health Journals.** Limits to consumer health journals.

Searching

LOCATING A SINGLE CITATION

Virtually anyone who uses MEDLINE will eventually need to retrieve a specific citation, perhaps simply to read the abstract or to verify a volume or page number. One easy way to retrieve a citation is to combine the author plus the first page plus the publication year.

Unfortunately, Ovid lacks a simple, elegant citation matcher like the one provided by PubMed. Whereas PubMed's Single Citation Matcher allows multiple terms to be added before running a search, Ovid's Search Fields page requires that the user search and combine terms separately. Consequently, searching for a citation using field tags is much more efficient.

Example: Locating a Specific Article

A user who is trying to locate an article by *C. M. Bloor* knows that the first page is 330 and that the publication date is 1988. (Remember that numeric fields such as page number need the numbers in quotation marks.) The search statement would then be *bloor cm.au and "330".pg and "1988".yr*.

The citation was found.

1. Roth DM. White FC. **Bloor** CM. Altered minimal coronary resistance to antegrade reflow after chronic coronary artery occlusion in swine. [Journal Article] *Circulation Research.* 63(2):**330**-9, **1988** Aug.
UI: 88282741

Abstract • Complete Reference

AUTHOR SEARCHING

An individual should keep the following things in mind when performing Author searches in Ovid MEDLINE: (a) MEDLINE does *not* understand first or middle names, so initials must be used; (b) sometimes authors use their middle initials, and sometimes they do not; (c) if the user is looking for articles *about* an author, he or she should add the tag *.pn* (personal name as subject) after the author's name (e.g., *shumway ne.pn.*); and (d) compound names can be entered without punctuation (e.g., *van der meer r*). The two main methods for running author searches are (a) a field-tag search on the command line and (b) the Author icon.

Command-Line Author Search

The easiest way to run an Ovid MEDLINE author search is to use command-line syntax. Simply append ".au." to the end of the author's name.

Example: Author Search With Last Name and the First Two Initials

To locate articles by Norman E. Shumway, enter *shumway ne.au.* on the command line. Click Perform Search.

Enter **Keyword** or phrase:	☑ Map Term to Subject Heading
shumway ne.au.	**Perform Search**

If the user does not have a middle initial or if an author sometimes used a middle initial and sometimes did not, truncate the author search after the first initial.

Example: Author Search With Last Name and First Initial (Any or No Middle Initial)

Locate articles by Norman Shumway. Type *shumway n$.au* on the Ovid command line. Click Perform Search.

Enter **Keyword** or phrase:	☑ Map Term to Subject Heading
shumway n$.au	**Perform Search**

Note that the second search retrieved more articles than the first.

#	Search History	Results	Display
1	shumway ne.au.	411	Display
2	shumway n$.au.	421	Display

● Saved Searches   ● Save Search History   ● Delete Searches

On occasions when only the last name of an author is known, type a space after the last name, then the truncation symbol ($), and then the field tag (.au).

Example: Locating an Author Using Only the Last Name

Locate articles by Shumway. Type *shumway $.au* on the Ovid command line. Be sure to leave a space between *shumway* and the dollar sign. Click Perform Search.

Enter **Keyword** or phrase:	☑ Map Term to Subject Heading
shumway $.au	**Perform Search**

Not surprisingly, the third search retrieved the most citations; however, it did include articles by other authors named Shumway.

#	Search History	Results	Display
1	shumway ne.au.	411	Display
2	shumway n$.au.	421	Display
3	shumway $.au.	630	Display

○ Saved Searches   ○ Save Search History   ○ Delete Searches

Author Icon

Ovid's author search icon allows searchers to browse through the author name index. This feature can come in handy when one is unsure of the spelling of an author's name.

Example: Misspelling an Author's Name

Locate articles by D. W. Hilgeman. Type *hilgeman dw* on the command line and then click the Author icon.

| Author | Title | Journal | Search Fields | Tools | Combine | Limit | Basic | Change Database | Logoff |

#	Search History	Results	Display
-	-	-	-

○ Saved Searches

Enter **Keyword** or phrase: ☑ Map Term to Subject Heading

`hilgeman dw`   **Perform Search**

The author's name appears to have a typo as no sign of a "D. W. Hilgeman" was found; however, a "D. W. Hilgemann" *was* located (**A**). Apparently, an "n" was missing in the original search. Click the checkbox next to "hilgemann dw" and then choose Perform Search (**B**).

Perform Search ◄ (**B**)   A Z Back in Index   🏠 Main Search Page   Forward in Index A Z

Enter a new start term: _____ Go

Choose from among the following index entries:

	Term	Postings
☐	hilgeman jl.au.	1
☐	hilgemann d.au.	1
☐	hilgemann dh.au.	1
☑	hilgemann dw.au.	40 ◄——— (**A**)

TOPIC SEARCHES

General Overview

As was mentioned earlier, the Ovid search interface is designed to make the most of a database's special strengths. When Map Term to Subject Heading is activated, Ovid leads the searcher through a MeSH search more effectively than does virtually any other MEDLINE search system. Depending on local configuration decisions, search terms are mapped to equivalent MeSH terms if any exist; the user is then shown to a list of relevant subheadings.

Integrating a Search into Ovid

Ovid MEDLINE can accommodate different types of searches quite nicely. The following search examples demonstrate how search terms can be integrated into Ovid MEDLINE using MeSH, subheadings, and search limits.

Examples: Review Articles on the Etiology of Fevers of Unknown Origin in Children. A user is looking for *review articles* on the *etiology* of *fevers of unknown origin* in *children.*

Fevers of Unknown Origin	Phrase gets mapped to the MeSH Fever of Unknown Origin.
Etiology	After selection of the MeSH term, Ovid provides a list of subheadings that includes Etiology.
Children	Click on the Limit icon, go to the Age Groups menu, and select All Child.
Review articles	Click on the Limit icon, go to the Publication Types menu, and select Review.

Example: Epidemiologic Studies on Atopic Dermatitis in Core Clinical Journals.

Atopic Dermatitis	Phrase is mapped to the MeSH Dermatitis, Atopic.
Epidemiology	After selection of the MeSH term, Ovid provides a list of subheadings that includes Epidemiology.
Core Clinical Journals	Click on the Limit icon, then go to the Journal Subset menu and select AIM Journals.

NOTE: Trying to figure out which part of the search goes where can be tricky. One shortcut is to locate a couple of relevant citations; display them in the Complete Reference format; see how they have been indexed; and then plug in the appropriate MeSH terms, subheadings, and publication types.

Developing a Search Strategy

The choice of a particular MEDLINE search strategy usually involves the following three factors: knowledge of the search system; time available for searching; and required depth or inclusiveness of the search. (See "Elements of an Effective Search" in Chapter 2).

For example, if a user needs to locate quickly a small number of articles on the treatment of meconium aspiration, he or she could select Ovid's Title search icon, enter *meconium aspiration*, and click Perform Search. It is simple and fast, and it can often retrieve a small number of highly relevant citations.

On the other hand, if the user plans to write a review article on gestational diabetes, he or she might want to run a MeSH plus free-text search. This search might be fairly complicated, and it may take some time to create, but a significant percentage of the journal literature on the subject will probably be retrieved.

The four Ovid MEDLINE search strategies discussed below are easily adaptable to the ever-fluctuating variables of skill, time, and inclusiveness. Each strategy includes commentary on when to use it, when to be careful, how it works, and sample search examples using screen shots. The strategies are listed *roughly* in the order of ease of use.

Strategy 1: Title Search

Strategy 2: Medical Subject Headings (MeSH)

Strategy 3: MeSH Plus Free Text

Strategy 4: Multifile

Search Strategy 1: Title Search

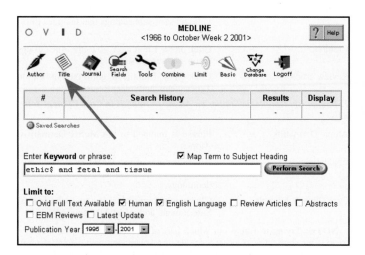

Advantages. It is fast, and it has high relevance. It is a great starting point for more complex strategies; this is one of the author's favorites.

Disadvantages. This strategy is definitely not comprehensive.

When to use. Title searches offer an effective strategy (a personal favorite) for identifying a couple of highly relevant articles quickly. Perhaps more important, a well-designed title search is one of the best ways to lay the groundwork for a more sophisticated and comprehensive search (see "Strategy 3: Medical Subject Headings Plus Free Text").

When to be careful. This is not a comprehensive search strategy; rather it is meant to pull up a small number of citations quickly.

How it works. This strategy is simple. If an author uses a title that includes the user's search terms, the chances are excellent that that citation is *extremely* relevant to the search. After all, titles often succinctly express the central themes of the article.

Keep in mind. Using terms that one could reasonably expect to find in the title of the article is important (e.g., *PET scans* versus *positron emission tomography scans*). Also, the searcher should make frequent use of truncation and synonyms.

Title Search Examples

Example: Management of Otitis Media. The user needs a couple of articles that discuss the *management of otitis media*. The search should be limited to Human studies, English, and 1995 to 2001 (**A**). Type in *manage$ and otitis media*. Select the search limits and then click the Title icon (**B**).

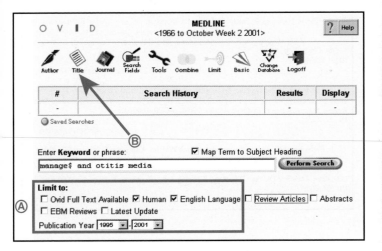

The search retrieved 61 citations. Click the Display icon to view the results.

Several citations appear relevant.

☐ 3. Ryan R. Harkness P. Fowler S. Topham J. **Manage**ment of paediatric **otitis media** with effusion in the UK: a survey conducted with the guidance of the Clinical Effectiveness Unit at the Royal College of Surgeons of England. [Journal Article] *Journal of Laryngology & Otology. 115(6):475-8, 2001 Jun.*
UI: 21322545

Abstract • Complete Reference

☐ 4. Hoberman A. Paradise JL. Acute **otitis media**: diagnosis and **manage**ment in the year 2000. [erratum appears in Pediatr Ann 2000 Dec;29(12):742]. [Review] [43 refs] [Journal Article. Review. Review, Tutorial] *Pediatric Annals. 29(10):609-20, 2000 Oct.*
UI: 20510698

Complete Reference

☐ 5. Pichichero ME. Reiner SA. Brook I. Gooch WM 3rd. Yamauchi T. Jenkins SG. Sher L. Controversies in the medical **management** of persistent and recurrent acute **otitis media**. Recommendations of a clinical advisory committee. [Guideline. Journal Article. Practice Guideline] *Annals of Otology, Rhinology, & Laryngology - Supplement. 183:1-12, 2000 Aug.*
UI: 20417606

Abstract • Complete Reference

Example: Complications of Epidural Anesthesia. To locate articles about the complications of epidural anesthesia, the user should limit the search to Human, English, and 1995 to 2001 (**A**). Type *complicat$ and epidural and anesthesia* on the command line. Click the Title icon (**B**).

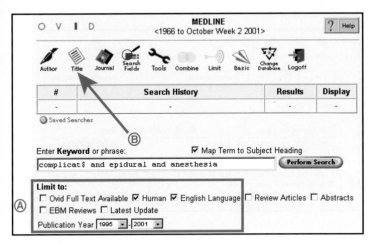

Ovid retrieved 11 citations, several of which are relevant. A more comprehensive search could include MeSH terms and subheadings, as the next example illustrates.

Results of your search: **limit 1 to (human and english language and yr=1995-2001)**
Citations displayed: **1-10** of 11
Go to Record: [1] (Go)   Citation Manager • Help • Logoff
Customize Display Reset Display

☐ 1. Horlocker TT. **Complications** of spinal and **epidural anesthesia**. [Review] [59 refs] [Journal Article. Review. Review, Academic] *Anesthesiology Clinics of North America. 18(2):461-85, 2000 Jun.*
UI: 20390688
                                                          Abstract • Complete Reference

☐ 2. Tang WM. Chiu KY. Silent compartment syndrome **complicating** total knee arthroplasty: continuous **epidural anesthesia** masked the pain. [Journal Article] *Journal of Arthroplasty. 15(2):241-3, 2000 Feb.*
UI: 20170368
                                                          Abstract • Complete Reference

☐ 3. Horlocker TT. Wedel DJ. Neurologic **complications** of spinal and **epidural anesthesia**. [Review] [80 refs] [Journal Article. Review. Review, Tutorial] *Regional **Anesthesia** & Pain Medicine. 25(1):83-98, 2000 Jan-Feb.*
UI: 20123644
                                                          Complete Reference

Example: Ovarian Cancer, Tamoxifen, and Breast Cancer Are there recent articles that report on ovarian cancer in women who take tamoxifen to prevent or treat breast cancer? Limit to English, Human, and 1998 to 2002 (**A**).

Type *tamoxifen and ovar$ and breast* onto the command line. Click the Title icon (**B**).

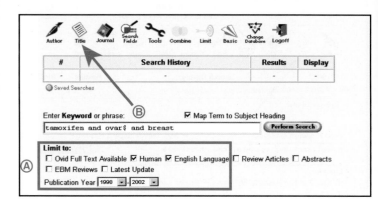

The search retrieved eight citations (**C**).

#	Search History	Results	Display
1	(tamoxifen and ovar$ and breast).ti.	28	Display
2	limit 1 to (human and english language and yr=1998-2002)	8	Display

Saved Searches   Save Search History   Delete Searches

Title searches can quickly retrieve high relevance citations that can form the basis for other, more comprehensive searches (see "Strategy 3: Medical Subject Headings Plus Free Text"). For example, to locate citations similar to the one listed below, start by clicking on the Complete Reference link (**D**) to display the citation's MeSH terms.

☐ 7. Cohen I. Bernheim J. Fishman A. Shapira J. Tepper R. Beyth Y. Cordoba M. Yigael D. Altaras MM.
Estrogen and progesterone receptors in benign **ovar**ian tumors of menopausal **breast** cancer patients treated with **tamoxifen**. [Journal Article] *Gynecologic & Obstetric Investigation. 46(2):116-22, 1998 Aug.*
UI: 98369030

Abstract • Complete Reference

Several MeSH/subheading combinations look particularly relevant, including, Breast Neoplasms/Drug Therapy (**A**), Ovarian Neoplasms/Chemically Induced (**B**), and Tamoxifen/Adverse Effects (**C**) (see "Strategy 2: Searching With Medical Subject Headings"). The MeSH terms could then be used in a new, more comprehensive search.

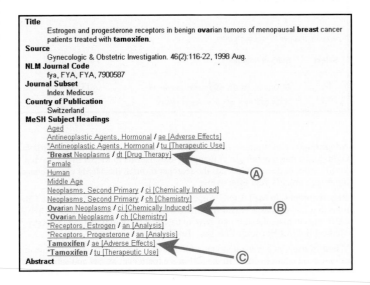

Title
Estrogen and progesterone receptors in benign **ovar**ian tumors of menopausal **breast** cancer patients treated with **tamoxifen**.
Source
Gynecologic & Obstetric Investigation. 46(2):116-22, 1998 Aug.
NLM Journal Code
fya, FYA, FYA, 7900587
Journal Subset
Index Medicus
Country of Publication
Switzerland
MeSH Subject Headings
Aged
Antineoplastic Agents, Hormonal / ae [Adverse Effects]
*Antineoplastic Agents, Hormonal / tu [Therapeutic Use]
*Breast Neoplasms / dt [Drug Therapy]
Female
Human
Middle Age
Neoplasms, Second Primary / ci [Chemically Induced]
Neoplasms, Second Primary / ch [Chemistry]
Ovarian Neoplasms / ci [Chemically Induced]
*Ovarian Neoplasms / ch [Chemistry]
*Receptors, Estrogen / an [Analysis]
*Receptors, Progesterone / an [Analysis]
Tamoxifen / ae [Adverse Effects]
*Tamoxifen / tu [Therapeutic Use]
Abstract

Search Strategy 2: Searching with Medical Subject Headings

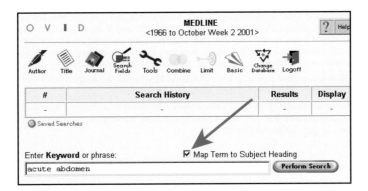

Advantages. This strategy is known for its high relevance and high retrieval. Ovid does a much better job of mapping search terms to MeSH than PubMed's MeSH browser does. Ovid leads the searcher through the MeSH plus subheading search process very effectively.

Disadvantages. In MEDLINE, some citations are inconsistently indexed. Citations in some databases (e.g., PREMEDLINE) lack MeSH terms. If Ovid MEDLINE fails to map, the user may have to try free-text searching (see "Strategy 3: Medical Subject Headings Plus Free Text").

When to use. An excellent strategy for searches that go beyond "give me one or two good citations fast." In the author's experience, MeSH and subheadings provide excellent results of moderate to high relevancy. If the search retrieves too much, whittling down the number of citations with Ovid's various search limits (e.g., review articles, date restrictions) is easy.

When to be careful. Enter terms individually. For example, do not type *ectopic pregnancy and methotrexate* on one line. Instead, type *ectopic pregnancy*, click Perform Search, and select the MeSH term, subheadings, and so on. Then enter the second term, *methotrexate*, click Perform Search, and select the MeSH term and subheadings. Combine the two search sets with *and*. If the terms fail to map to MeSH terms, the user might need to retrieve a couple of relevant articles (e.g., with a title search) and then check how they have been indexed. If no MeSH terms exist for the topic, the searcher should use free-text searching.

How it works. When Map Term to Subject Heading is checked, Ovid attempts to map the search terms to their equivalent MeSH terms.

Keep in mind. One of Ovid's advantages is its ability to integrate a database's special features (e.g., MeSH, subheadings) into the search process smoothly. Be sure to take advantage of this.

Medical Subject Heading Search Examples

Example: Review Articles on Hepatitis C. When looking for recent review articles on treatment for hepatitis C, type *hepatitis C* on the command line, make sure that the Map Term to Subject Heading checkbox is clicked, and then click Perform Search.

Ovid displays a Mapping Display screen with the MeSH Hepatitis C already preselected. At this point, the user could supplement the search with a free-text search of the term *hepatitis C*. Scope provides additional information about the MeSH term (e.g., definition, indexing history). Because so much has been written about hepatitis C, using Focus (**A**) to limit the search to articles in which Hepatitis C is a major theme might be a good idea. Click Continue (**B**).

125

NOTE: Depending on how Ovid MEDLINE is configured at a particular institution, an option labeled Explode may appear. Explode will automatically search narrower MeSH terms. If this option does not appear, then Explode has almost certainly been configured to occur automatically.

Ovid now shows all the available subheadings for the MeSH Hepatitis C. Because the user is interested in treatment, several choices are available. Select Diet Therapy and Drug Therapy (**A**), Therapy and Surgery (**B**), and Prevention & Control (**C**). Click Continue (**D**).

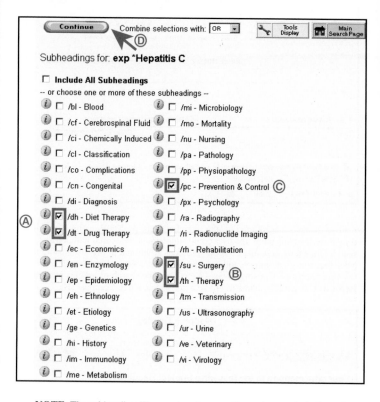

NOTE: The subheading Therapy is rather peculiar and, as such, is deserving of a bit of clarification. By itself, Therapy is considered to include therapies that *are not* drug therapy, diet therapy, radiotherapy, or surgery. It applies to articles that discuss general, unspecified, or multiple therapies. Unlike PubMed, selecting Therapy in Ovid will *not* automatically include its narrower subheadings (e.g., diet therapy, drug therapy).

The search retrieved more than 3,000 citations. Now the user must restrict the search using search limits. Limit the search to Human, English Language, Review Articles, and 1998 through 2001 (**A**). Click Perform Search (**B**).

Many of the retrieved citations seem to be highly relevant.

☑ 3. Lemon MD. Meade F. The basics of new treatment for chronic **hepatitis** C. [Review] [9 refs] [Journal Article. Review. Review, Tutorial] *South Dakota Journal of Medicine.* 54(8):303-4, 2001 Aug.
UI: 21415181

Complete Reference

☐ 4. Bockhold KM. Who's afraid of **hepatitis** C? [see comments]. [Review] [18 refs] [Journal Article. Review. Review, Tutorial] *American Journal of Nursing.* 100(5):26-31; quiz 32, 2000 May.
UI: 20282571

Complete Reference • **Ovid Full Text**

☑ 5. Wang QM. Heinz BA. Recent advances in prevention and treatment of **hepatitis** C virus infections. [Review] [159 refs] [Journal Article. Review. Review, Tutorial] *Progress in Drug Research.* Spec No:79-110, 2001.
UI: 21430206

Abstract • Complete Reference

☐ 6. Asmar BI. Abdel-Haq NM. Antiviral therapy: respiratory infections, chronic **hepatitis**. [Review] [34 refs] [Journal Article. Review. Review, Tutorial] *Indian Journal of Pediatrics.* 68(7):635-9, 2001 Jul.
UI: 21411037

Abstract • Complete Reference

☑ 7. Kozlowski A. Charles SA. Harris JM. Development of pegylated interferons for the treatment of chronic **hepatitis** C. [Review] [46 refs] [Journal Article. Review. Review, Tutorial] *Biodrugs.* 15(7):419-29, 2001.
UI: 21411405

Abstract • Complete Reference

Example: Quality of Life Following Liver Transplantation. *Do not* combine all the search terms in one statement; instead, type *quality of life* onto the command line and click Perform Search.

As with the previous search, the searcher could choose Focus. However, *quality of life + liver transplantation* should generate far fewer citations than *treatment of Hepatitis C*, so this search should *not* be restricted to Focus, which would introduce the risk of missing something relevant. Instead, click Continue.

Select the checkbox next to Include All Subheadings and click Continue.

The search retrieved almost 30,000 citations. Type *liver transplantation* on the command line and click Perform Search.

At the Mapping Display screen, click Continue.

Attempting to pick out the best subheadings for this particular search (psychology? rehabilitation?) is difficult. Play it safe and choose Include All Subheadings (**A**). Click Continue (**B**).

Combine the two searches by typing *1 and 2* on the command line. Select Human, English, Review Articles, and 1995 through 2001 as the search limits (**C**). Click Perform Search (**D**).

Several appear to be right on target.

☐ 4. Bravata DM. Keeffe EB. Quality of life and employment after liver transplantation. [Review] [20 refs] [Journal Article. Review. Review, Tutorial] *Liver Transplantation*. 7(11 Suppl 1):S119-23, 2001 Nov.
UI: 11689784

Abstract • Complete Reference

☐ 5. Adam SJ. Palliative care for patients with a failed liver transplant. [Review] [18 refs] [Journal Article. Review. Review, Tutorial] *Intensive & Critical Care Nursing*. 16(6):396-402, 2000 Dec.
UI: 11091471

Abstract • Complete Reference

☐ 6. Heitkemper M. Jarrett M. Kurashige EM. Carithers R. Chronic hepatitis C. Implications for health-related quality of life. [see comments.] [Review] [42 refs] [Journal Article. Review. Review, Tutorial] *Gastroenterology Nursing*. 24(4):169-7 quiz 176-7, 2001 Jul-Aug.
UI: 11848000

Abstract • Complete Reference • Ovid Full Tex

☐ 7. Habib A. Bond WM. Heuman DM. Long-term management of cirrhosis. Appropriate supportive care is both critical and difficult. [Review] [27 refs] [Journal Article. Review. Review, Tutorial] *Postgraduate Medicine*. 109(3):101-13, 2001 Mar
UI: 11265349

Abstract • Complete Reference

☐ 8. Kim WR. Dickson ER. Timing of liver transplantation. [Review] [32 refs] [Journal Article. Review. Review, Tutorial] Seminars in *Liver* Disease. 20(4):451-64, 2000.
UI: 11200415

Abstract • Complete Reference

Example: Sensitivity and Specificity of Enzyme-Linked Immunosorbent Pulmonary Assay (ELISA) in Tuberculosis.

NOTE: Quotation marks must be used around *"sensitivity and specificity"* to ensure that Ovid sees these terms as a phrase. Otherwise, Ovid will combine the searches—one on sensitivity and the other on specificity.

Type *"sensitivity and specificity."* Click Perform Search.

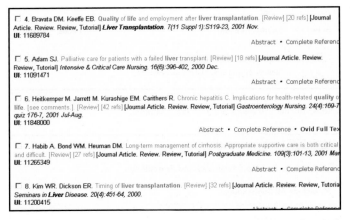

131

Ovid displays the MeSH term *sensitivity and specificity*. Click Continue.

Continue ←			
Select	**Subject Heading**	**Focus**	**Scope**
☑	"Sensitivity and Specificity"	☐	*i*
☐	"sensitivity and specificity".mp. *search as Keyword*		

Choose Include All Subheadings. Click Continue.

Continue ←

Subheadings for: **exp Sensitivity and Specificity**

☑ **Include All Subheadings**
-- or choose one or more of these subheadings --
i ☐ /st - Standards

Type *pulmonary tuberculosis* onto the command line. Click Perform Search.

Enter **Keyword** or phrase: ☑ Map Term to Subject Heading

pulmonary tuberculosis   **Perform Search**

Ovid retrieves the MeSH Tuberculosis, Pulmonary. Click Continue.

Continue ←			
Select	**Subject Heading**	**Focus**	**Scope**
☑	Tuberculosis, Pulmonary	☐	*i*
☐	pulmonary tuberculosis.mp. *search as Keyword*		

132

Choose Diagnosis from the subheadings menu (**A**). Click Continue (**B**).

Type *elisa* onto the command line and click Perform Search.

Ovid retrieves the MeSH Enzyme-Linked Immunosorbent Assay. Click Continue.

Choose Include All Subheadings. Click Continue.

Combining the three sets retrieves 63 citations. Click on the Limits icon.

Choose Human, English, All Child, and 1995 through 2001. Click Limit Search.

This search strategy retrieved nine citations.

#	Search History	Results	Display
2	exp Tuberculosis, Pulmonary/di [Diagnosis]	6274	Display
3	exp Enzyme-Linked Immunosorbent Assay/	56731	Display
4	1 and 2 and 3	63	Display
5	limit 4 to (human and english language and all child <0 to 18 years> and yr=1995-2001)	9	Display

Again, a fair number of these citations seem relevant.

☑ 1. Pottumarthy S. Wells VC. Morris AJ. A comparison of seven tests for serological diagnosis of tuberculosis. [Clinical Trial. Journal Article] *Journal of Clinical Microbiology.* *38(6):2227-31, 2000 Jun.*
UI: 20295098

Abstract • Complete Reference

☑ 2. Simonney N. Bourrillon A. Lagrange PH. Analysis of circulating immune complexes (CICs) in childhood tuberculosis: levels of specific antibodies to glycolipid antigens **and** relationship with serum antibodies. [Clinical Trial. Controlled Clinical Trial. Journal Article] *International Journal of Tuberculosis & Lung Disease. 4(2):152-60, 2000 Feb.*
UI: 20155786

Abstract • Complete Reference

☑ 3. Swaminathan S. Umadevi P. Shantha S. Radhakrishnan A. Datta M. Sero diagnosis of tuberculosis in children using two ELISA kits. [Clinical Trial. Journal Article] *Indian Journal of Pediatrics. 66(6):837-42, 1999 Nov-Dec.*
UI: 20258483

Abstract • Complete Reference

☑ 4. Sant'Anna CC. Ferreira MA. Fonseca LS. Evaluation of a serological method (ELISA) for the diagnosis of **pulmonary** tuberculosis in children. [Letter] *International Journal of Tuberculosis & Lung Disease. 3(8):744, 1999 Aug.*
UI: 99387869

Complete Reference

135

Search Strategy 3: Medical Subject Headings
Plus Title or Free Text

| O V I D | MEDLINE <1966 to October Week 2 2001> | ? Help |

| Author | Title | Journal | Search Fields | Tools | Combine | Limit | Basic | Change Database | Logoff |

#	Search History	Results	Display
-	-	-	-

Saved Searches

Enter **Keyword** or phrase: ☑ Map Term to Subject Heading

`exp acute abdomen/di or (diagn$ and acute abdomen)`   **Perform Search**

Limit to:
☐ Ovid Full Text Available ☐ Human ☑ English Language ☐ Review Articles ☐ Abstracts
☐ EBM Reviews ☐ Latest Update
Publication Year [1995 ▾] - [2001 ▾]

Advantages. Supplementing MeSH with a free-text or title search is often a highly effective strategy for more comprehensive searching.

Disadvantages. This strategy can be more complicated and can take more time than others.

When to use. When a user wants to run a search that strikes a balance between moderate to high recall and moderate to high precision, the author typically recommends a combination MeSH plus Title search; if precision is less important than recall (or if the topic is not well covered in the literature), a broader MeSH plus Free-Text Search is recommended.

When to be careful. This strategy can take longer than other strategies.

How it works. A supplemental title or free-text search can retrieve citations that have been missed because some of the search terms lack equivalent MeSH terms or because they were inconsistently indexed.

Keep in mind. If the supplemental title search retrieves too few citations, switch to a supplemental free-text search.

MeSH Plus Title or Free-Text Search Examples

Example: Complications of Endoscopic Carpal Tunnel Release. Start by running a title search on some key terms. The goal is to locate some relevant citations, look at their MeSH terms, and then search the most relevant. Although Ovid could easily map these particular search terms to MeSH, this example is good practice for occasions when Ovid *cannot* map successfully. Type *complicat$ and carpal tunnel and endoscop$* on the command line. Click the Title icon (**A**).

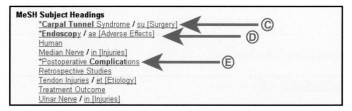

Locate some relevant citations and click Complete Reference (**B**) to view their MeSH terms.

☐ 3. Palmer AK. Toivonen DA. Complications of endoscopic and open carpal tunnel release. [see comments]. [Journal Article] *Journal of Hand Surgery - American Volume.* *24(3):561-5, 1999 May.* **UI**: 99284428

Abstract • Complete Reference (**B**)

Carpal Tunnel Syndrome/su [Surgery] (**C**), Endoscopy/ae [Adverse Effects] (**D**), and Postoperative Complications (**E**) appear extremely relevant. Return to the main search page and plug them in.

MeSH Subject Headings
  *Carpal Tunnel Syndrome / su [Surgery] ◀——— (**C**)
  *Endoscopy / ae [Adverse Effects] ◀——— (**D**)
  Human
  Median Nerve / in [Injuries]
  *Postoperative Complications ◀——— (**E**)
  Retrospective Studies
  Tendon Injuries / et [Etiology]
  Treatment Outcome
  Ulnar Nerve / in [Injuries]

Enter *carpal tunnel syndrome* on the command line. Click Perform Search.

Enter **Keyword** or phrase: ☑ Map Term to Subject Heading
carpal tunnel syndrome   **Perform Search**

137

Click Continue.

Select	Subject Heading	Focus	Scope
☑	**Carpal Tunnel Syndrome**	☐	ⓘ
☐	carpal tunnel syndrome.mp. *search as Keyword*		

Choose the subheading Surgery (**A**). Click Continue (**B**).

- ⓘ ☐ /ep - Epidemiology
- ⓘ ☐ /eh - Ethnology
- ⓘ ☐ /et - Etiology
- ⓘ ☐ /ge - Genetics
- ⓘ ☐ /hi - History
- ⓘ ☐ /im - Immunology
- ⓘ ☑ /su - Surgery
- ⓘ ☐ /th - Therapy
- ⓘ ☐ /us - Ultrasonography
- ⓘ ☐ /ve - Veterinary
- ⓘ ☐ /vi - Virology

Enter *postoperative complications* on the command line. Click Perform Search.

Enter **Keyword** or phrase: ☑ Map Term to Subject Heading

postoperative complications **Perform Search**

Click Continue.

Select	Subject Heading	Focus	Scope
☑	**Postoperative Complications**	☐	ⓘ
☐	postoperative complications.mp. *search as Keyword*		

Click Include All Subheadings.

Subheadings for: **exp Postoperative Complications**

☑ **Include All Subheadings**
-- or choose one or more of these subheadings --

Enter *endoscopy* on the command line. Click Perform Search.

> Enter **Keyword** or phrase: ☑ Map Term to Subject Heading
> endoscopy
> (Perform Search) ⬅

Make sure Endoscopy is selected, and then click Continue.

Select	Subject Heading	Focus	Scope
☑	**ENDOSCOPY**	☐	ⓘ
☐	ENDOSCOPY, DIGESTIVE SYSTEM	☐	ⓘ
☐	ENDOSCOPY, GASTROINTESTINAL	☐	ⓘ
☐	endoscopy.mp. *search as Keyword*		

(Continue) ⬅

Select */ae—Adverse Effects* (**A**) and */ct—Contraindications* (**B**). The two will be combined with *OR*, and the searcher will get either *Endoscopy/Adverse Effects* OR *Endoscopy/Contraindications*.

> Subheadings for: **exp ENDOSCOPY**
>
> ☐ **Include All Subheadings**
> -- or choose one or more of these subheadings --
> ⓘ ☑ /ae - Adverse Effects ⬅   ⓘ ☐ /nu - Nursing Ⓐ
> ⓘ ☐ /cl - Classification   ⓘ ☐ /px - Psychology
> ⓘ ☑ /ct - Contraindications ⬅ ⓘ ☐ /rh - Rehabilitation Ⓑ

Before combining searches, run one more title search. The idea is to catch citations that might have been inconsistently indexed (e.g., citations where the indexer might have added the MeSH Endoscopy but might have left off the subheadings Adverse Effects or Contraindications). The supplemental title search is a bit broader than the original as it includes the word *adverse* as well as *complicat$*.

Enter *(adverse or complicat$) and carpal tunnel and endoscop$* in the command line. Click the Title icon.

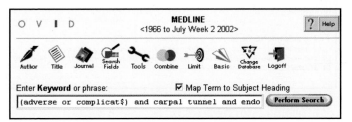

Whew! This search is almost done. The sets (**A**) can now be combined. In parentheses, first combine sets 2, 3, and 4 using the Boolean operator *AND*. Then combine these sets with the supplementary title search using the operator *OR*.

Enter *(2 and 3 and 4) or 5* on the command line. Limit the search to English and 1995 through 2001 (**B**). Click Perform Search (**C**).

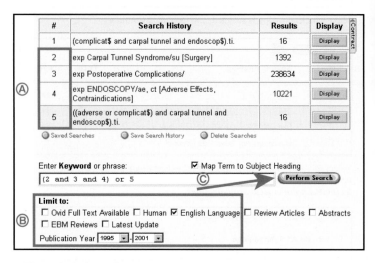

The results look excellent.

☐ 1. Muller LP. Rudig L. Degreif J. Rommens PM. Endoscopic carpal tunnel release: results with special consideration to possible complications. [Review] [47 refs] [Journal Article. Review. Review of Reported Cases] *Knee Surgery, Sports Traumatology, Arthroscopy. 8(3):166-72, 2000.*
UI: 20339643

Abstract • Complete Reference

☐ 2. Kasdan ML. Complications of endoscopic and open carpal tunnel release. [letter; comment]. [Comment. Letter] *Journal of Hand Surgery - American Volume. 25(1):185, 2000 Jan.*
UI: 20111252

Complete Reference

☐ 3. Palmer AK. Toivonen DA. Complications of endoscopic and open carpal tunnel release. [see comments]. [Journal Article] *Journal of Hand Surgery - American Volume. 24(3):561-5, 1999 May.*
UI: 99284428

Abstract • Complete Reference

☐ 4. Boeckstyns ME. Sorensen AI. Does endoscopic carpal tunnel release have a higher rate of complications than open carpal tunnel release? An analysis of published series. [Journal Article. Meta-Analysis] *Journal of Hand Surgery - British Volume. 24(1):9-15, 1999 Feb.*
UI: 99204871

Abstract • Complete Reference

Search Strategy 4: Multifile Search

Advantages. Searching multiple databases can significantly increase search retrieval. Ovid also provides a duplicate citation feature, as well as access to several powerful EBM databases if the user has access to them.

Disadvantages. Because different databases often have different indexing terms and vocabularies, this search strategy is potentially complex and time-consuming.

When to use. If the user subscribes to multiple Ovid databases, he or she should be sure to take advantage of the multifile search feature. If the user is not sure which database is best for a particular topic, choose several and see which database produces the most hits or consult with a medical librarian. If the user needs to run a particularly comprehensive search, selecting up to five databases

141

for simultaneous searching is possible. The author finds that multifile searching is particularly useful with Ovid's EBMR collection.

When to be careful. Whenever searching multiple databases, the user must take into account differences in indexing terms and subject vocabularies. For example, the Cochrane Controlled Trials Register contains some citations indexed with MeSH terms, some with EMBASE subject headings, and some with no subject headings at all. Also, search limits that are available in some databases may be ignored in others (e.g., the Protocols limit *does not* apply to MEDLINE). The more a user knows about a database before searching it, the better.

Keep in mind. Some of the databases may need to be searched individually to take full advantage of their respective search features.

Multifile Search Examples

Example: Vitamin C in the Treatment or Prevention of the Common Cold.
The EBMR databases are particularly effective for searches looking at the effectiveness of treatment X on disease Y. So, in addition to MEDLINE and Pre-MEDLINE, the search could include the ACP Journal Club, the Cochrane Database of Systematic Reviews, and the Cochrane Controlled Trials Register. Use the "Select more than one database to search" tab to choose the five databases.

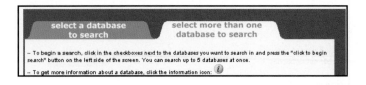

The relatively small size of these collections (when compared with MEDLINE) means that one can search more broadly with less chance of being overwhelmed by too many citations. Thus, a free-text search is often the search tool of choice for the EBMR databases. The fact that many of these databases lack MeSH makes a free-text search even more important. The search therefore combines MeSH (for citations indexed with subject headings) and free text (for those with MeSH indexing).

Start by locating the MeSH terms. As Map Term to Subject Heading is not an option in multifile searching, a bootstrapping strategy that uses a title search can be employed.

Type *vitamin c and common cold* on the command line and click the Title search icon.

Scroll down a bit and click the "MEDLINE" link. (MEDLINE citations will have MeSH terms.)

Locate a relevant citation and then click on Complete Reference to view the MeSH terms. Ascorbic Acid (**A**) and Common Cold (**B**) are the two MeSH that should be chosen. Go back to the main search page and plug them in.

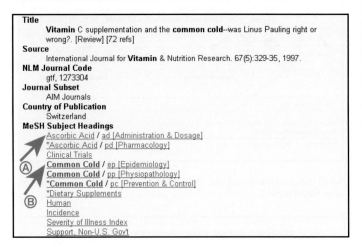

Since the automatic MeSH mapping is turned off, search the MeSH terms directly using the Explode command. If Explode is used, the search will retrieve the MeSH and any narrower MeSH terms as well. Type *exp ascorbic acid and exp common cold*.

Enter **Keyword** or phrase:

exp ascorbic acid and exp common cold

(**Perform Search**)

Now supplement the MeSH search with a free-text search to retrieve citations from databases that are not indexed with MeSH. An almost infinite number of possibilities exist for constructing this part of the search; how a particular seacher structures it depends on how comprehensive he or she wants the search to be.

Type *(ascorbic acid or vitamin c) and (cold$ or respiratory)* and click Perform Search.

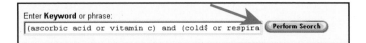

Enter **Keyword** or phrase:

(ascorbic acid or vitamin c) and (cold$ or respira

(**Perform Search**)

Now combine set 2 with set 3 using the Boolean operator *OR*. Restricting the search to English (**A**) and 1998 to 2002 (**B**) should provide a reasonable number of citations. Click Perform Search (**C**).

The search retrieved 133 citations. Click Remove Duplicates.

Ovid displays a duplicate deletion page with a variety of options. Database Preference lets searchers indicate a preference for a particular database citation format (e.g., MEDLINE citations contain more indexing information than identical citations from PsycINFO). Field Preference allows the user to indicate whether citations with a preferred feature (e.g., indexing terms such as MeSH) should be preferred to identical citations without that feature. Set as desired and Click Continue.

Edit Deduping Preferences

Field Preferences	Database Preferences	
○ Has Abstract	First Database	MEDLINE
● Has Full Text	Second Database	ACP Journal Club
○ Has Index Terms	Third Database	CCTR
○ No Field Preference	Fourth Database	Cochrane Database
	Fifth Database	Pre-MEDLINE

Hints:

- Use the Field and Database Preferences options to determine how the Ovid system will dedup your set.
- Select a single Field Preference. This Field Preference will be applied first in determining which records to keep versus which records to reject when duplicates are found.
- Rank the databases based on which record format you prefer. Your Database Preferences will be applied in the order chosen, after your Field Preference criteria.
- Once your set has been deduped, you will have an opportunity to review the duplicate records.

The following screen indicates that the search set contained zero duplicates.

No duplicates were detected!

Several of the citations look good.

☐ 1. *EBM Reviews - Cochrane Controlled Trials Register* Gorton HC; Jarvis K **The** effectiveness of vitamin C in **preventing** and **relieving the symptoms** of **virus-induced** respiratory infections. [Clinical Trial. CCT. Journal Article] *Journal of Manipulative & Physiological Therapeutics. 22(8):530-3, 1999 Oct.*
Abstract • Complete Reference

☐ 2. *MEDLINE* **Douglas** RM. Chalker EB. Treacy B. Vitamin C for **preventing** and **treating the common cold.** [Review] [30 refs] [Journal Article. Review. Review, Academic] *Cochrane Database of Systematic Reviews [computer file]. (2):CD000980, 2000.*
UI: 20257659
Abstract • Complete Reference

☐ 3. *MEDLINE* **Hemila** H. Vitamin C supplementation and **common cold symptoms**: problems with inaccurate reviews. [Review] [69 refs] [Journal Article. Review. Review, Tutorial] *Nutrition. 12(11-12):804-9, 1996 Nov-Dec.*
UI: 97129600
Abstract • Complete Reference

Section 3: Post-Search Data Management

CITATION MANAGER

The primary tool for printing, saving, and downloading citations in Ovid is the Citation Manager, which offers searchers an intuitive and compact set of tools for managing citations.

Citation Manager: Display, Print, Save, or Email Citations ↓			
Citations	**Fields**	**Citation Format**	**Action**
◉ Selected Citations ○ All on this page ○ All in this set (1-107) and/or Range:	○ Citation (Title,Author,Source) ◉ Citation + Abstract ○ Citation + Abstract + Subject Headings ○ Complete Reference Select Fields	◉ Ovid ○ BRS/Tagged ○ Reprint/Medlars ○ Brief (Titles) Display ○ Direct Export ☐ Include Search History	Display Print Preview Email Save
Sort Keys			
Primary:	▼ Ascending ▼		
Secondary:	▼ Ascending ▼		

The Citation Manager is divided into the following five sections: Citations, Fields, Citation Format, Action, and Sort Keys.

Citations. The searcher can use this section to tell Ovid which citations he or she intends to print, e-mail, and so on.

Fields. The fields that are to be included with the citations can be indicated here. Select Fields allows the user to choose virtually *any* field from the citation.

Citation Format. The Ovid format is essentially a more structured and less compact version of the Brief (Titles) Display. The other formats, BRS/Tagged, Reprint/Medlars, and Direct Export, are designed for bibliographic management software, such as Endnote, ProCite, and Reference Manager (see "Using Citation Management Software"). An option exists for including the search history with the printed or downloaded citations.

Action. This option indicates what action should be taken with the citations. Display presents citations in the indicated format, and it also retains the citation's links (e.g., to abstracts and full text). The Print Preview button has the same function as Display, but it does remove the links. E-mail will allow the user to e-mail the citations, and Save will provide a vehicle for saving them to a file.

Sort Keys. These are used to change the order in which the citations are listed, either by author or by year.

PRINTING, SAVING OR DOWNLOADING, AND E-MAILING

Printing

Printing citations in Ovid is *extremely* simple.

Example: Printing a Search Set

Select All in this set, Citation + Abstract, and Brief (Titles) Display (compresses the size of the citations and saves paper). Click the Print Preview button.

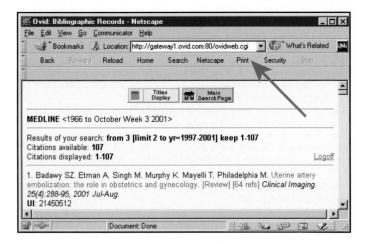

Once the citations are displayed, simply click on the Web browser's Print button.

Saving

Saving is almost as easy as printing.

Example: Saving a Search Set

Save all the citations in the search set; include abstracts, subject headings, and search history. Select the Ovid citation format. After making the selections, click Save.

When using a PC, the user should choose Windows Style Linefeeds. Click Continue.

Decide where to save the file, give it a name, and then click Save. Saving is then complete.

149

E-Mailing

Ovid makes e-mailing as easy as printing and saving.

Example: E-mail a Search Set

E-mail only the selected citations, including the abstracts, using the Ovid format. After making the appropriate selections, click E-mail.

Enter the e-mail address of the recipient, click the checkbox next to Include Search History, and click Send E-mail.

Ovid should confirm that the citations were e-mailed.

SAVING SEARCHES

Sometimes one wants to save a search temporarily for some reason (e.g., to eat lunch or to answer a page). Having the ability to save the search, run it automatically each time a database is updated, and then have the results sent via e-mail is convenient. For situations such as this, Ovid's marvelous save search features are the answer. The save options are as follows:

Temporarily. Save the search strategy for 24 hours or longer, depending on how Ovid is configured at a specific institution.

Permanently. This option saves a strategy until the user deletes it.

AutoAlert. This choice saves a strategy permanently and reruns it automatically. Any new citations added to the database that match this search profile will be sent via e-mail.

Example: Staying Current with a Topic

If a user is interested in articles that discuss methotrexate as a treatment for ectopic pregnancies, he or she will run a search, download some citations, and perhaps then import them into a citation management program (e.g., EndNote). To stay up-to-date, the user should save the search strategy by using AutoAlert (if it has been enabled at the particular institution). As new citations are added to the database, they will be compared with the stored search strategy and any matches will be sent to the user via e-mail. To do this, the user clicks Save Search History.

Choose *as an AutoAlert* and then scroll down a bit.

Enter a recipient e-mail address (more than one can be added), select the fields (in this case, Citation + Abstract + Subject Headings [**A**]), and indicate a citation format (e.g., Reprint/Medlars [**B**] to import the citations into a citation management program like EndNote). Click Save Search (**C**).

Ovid confirms that the search was saved. To view the saved search, the user clicks Saved Searches.

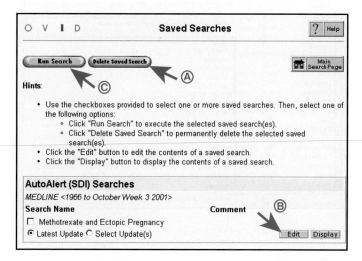

At this point, the user can delete (**A**), edit (**B**), or rerun (**C**) the saved search.

E-mail updates should begin to arrive within a week.

USING CITATION MANAGEMENT SOFTWARE

Citation management software, which is also known as reprint or bibliographic management software, is a terrific tool that can help one organize file cabinets full of article reprints or megabytes worth of downloaded Ovid citations. Even more amazing is the ability of these programs to format manuscript bibliographies quickly and easily. Simply select a bibliography style, click a button, and the in-text citations of the manuscript are instantly converted into a nicely formatted bibliography.

Below is a screen shot of an EndNote "library" of 22 imported PubMed citations. One of the citations has been opened.

Users can insert these citations into the text of a document (e.g., a Microsoft Word document) and then can create a bibliography from the citations in a wide range of bibliographic formats.

Although a detailed description of these programs is beyond the scope of this handbook, the next couple of pages illustrates techniques for downloading citations from Ovid and importing them into EndNote.

Importing

Ovid MEDLINE citations can be imported into EndNote (a) by searching Ovid MEDLINE from within EndNote (the downside of this approach is that the Ovid MEDLINE search interface is *significantly* more powerful than that which is provided by EndNote); (b) by downloading the citations in the BRS/Tagged or

Reprint/Medlars format and then importing them using EndNote's Import option; or (c) by choosing Direct Export, which, if it is configured properly, should drop the citations directly into EndNote.

Example: Importing Citations

After running a search, choose which citations to download, what fields should be included (MeSH provide additional search points within the EndNote library), and the display format Reprint/Medlars (**A**). Click Save (**B**).

Citation Manager: Display, Print, Save, or Email Citations ⬆			
Citations	**Fields**	**Citation Format**	**Action**
○ Selected Citations	○ Citation (Title,Author,Source)	○ Ovid	Display
○ All on this page	○ Citation + Abstract	○ BRS/Tagged	Print Preview
◉ All in this set (1-72)	◉ Citation + Abstract + Subject Headings	◉ Reprint/Medlars	Email
and/or Range:	○ Complete Reference	○ Brief (Titles) Display	Save
	Select Fields (A)	○ Direct Export	
		☐ Include Search History	
Sort Keys			
Primary:	- ▾	Ascending ▾	
Secondary:	- ▾	Ascending ▾	(B)

Choose Windows Style Linefeeds (**A**) when using a PC. Click Continue (**B**).

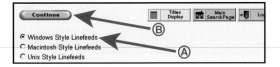

Be certain that the citations are saved with a .txt extension. This ensures that the citations are saved as plain text, which most citation management programs can import without any trouble.

Save As...	? ✕
Save in: 🗀 OVID Searches ▾ [⬆] [🗋] [▦] [▤]	
File name: mycites.txt	Save
Save as type: Plain Text (*.txt) ▾	Cancel

155

Next, be certain to indicate the source (e.g., Ovid) of the downloaded citations so that EndNote will recognize the unique Ovid MEDLINE format. In EndNote, choose Import Filters from the File pull-down menu and select Open Filters Manager. Select MEDLINE (Ovid).

Name	Information Provider
☐ MEDLINE (NLM)1	National Library of Medicine (NLM/Grateful Med)
☐ MEDLINE (NLM)2	
☐ MEDLINE (OCLC)	OCLC FirstSearch
☑ MEDLINE (OVID) ←	Ovid
☐ Medline (SP)	SilverPlatter

Import the saved Ovid records with the EndNote Import option. Find the file using the Choose File button. Select an Import Option; in this case, it is MEDLINE (Ovid). Choose Discard Duplicates to delete duplicate records. Click the Import button.

Import Data File:	mycites.txt [Choose File...]
Import Option:	MEDLINE (OVID) ▼
Duplicates:	Discard Duplicates ▼
Text Translation:	No Translation ▼
	[Import] [Cancel]

Seventy-one records were successfully imported into the EndNote library.

To insert citations into a document (e.g., an article manuscript), first select the desired citations.

Methotrexate2.enl

Author	Year	Title
Buster	2000	Current issues in medical management of ectopic pregnancy
Spitz	2000	Progesterone receptor modulators and progesterone antagonists in women's
Lipscomb	2000	Nonsurgical treatment of ectopic pregnancy
Barnhart	2000	An update on the medical treatment of ectopic pregnancy
Tulandi	2000	Evidence-based management of ectopic pregnancy
Buster	1999	Medical management of ectopic pregnancy
Fylstra	1999	Early diagnosis of ectopic pregnancy and treatment with methotrexate
Bruhat	1993	Endoscopic treatment of ectopic pregnancies

Showing 8 out of 8 references. ▼ Show Preview

Next, open a word processing program, such as Microsoft Word. When End-Note is installed, it adds features to the Word Tools pull-down menu. Thus, to insert the selected citations into a Word document, simply go to the Tools menu, select EndNote, and then click on Insert Selected Citation(s).

After inserting the citations into the document, choose a bibliography format from EndNote's enormous collection of bibliographic styles (e.g., *Nature Medicine*).

The following screen shot shows a fully formatted bibliography.

REFERENCES

1. Ovid home page. Available at: http://www.ovid.com/. Accessed May 2002.

APPENDIX A

Ovid's Evidence-Based Medicine Reviews Collection

The following descriptions were taken directly from Ovid's Field Guides. Quotation marks are omitted, but references for these guides appear at the end of Appendix A.

COCHRANE DATABASE OF SYSTEMATIC REVIEWS (1)

The Cochrane Database of Systematic Reviews (COCH) includes the full text of the regularly updated systematic reviews of the effects of health care that are prepared by the Cochrane Collaboration. The following two types of reviews are presented:

- Complete reviews: regularly updated Cochrane Reviews, prepared and maintained by Collaborative Review Groups.
- Protocols: protocols for reviews currently being prepared (all include an expected date of completion). Protocols are the background, objectives, and methods of reviews in preparation.

COCH is produced by the Cochrane Collaboration, an international network of individuals and institutions committed to preparing, maintaining, and disseminating systematic reviews of the effects of health care. In pursuing its aims, the Cochrane Collaboration is guided by the following six principles: collaboration, building on people's existing enthusiasm and interests, minimizing duplication of effort, avoidance of bias, remaining up-to-date, and ensuring access.

Each issue of COCH contains new and updated reviews and protocols. COCH is unlike other 'journal' or 'serial' publications in that, once a review is published, it will appear in every issue thereafter. Because of this, each Review or Protocol includes a section about how to cite that document if needed.

COCHRANE CONTROLLED TRIALS REGISTER (2)

Cochrane Controlled Trials Register (CCTR) is a bibliographic database of definitive controlled trials. These controlled trials have been identified by the distinguished contributors to the Cochrane Collaboration. They and others, as part of an international effort to search the world's health care journals (and other sources of information) systematically, have combined results to create an unbiased source of data for systematic reviews.

Because existing bibliographic databases have been shown to be inadequate for the identification of all relevant studies, the Cochrane Collaboration embarked upon this formidable task in cooperation with the National Library of Medicine (NLM) in Washington, D.C. (United States), who produces MEDLINE, and Reed Elsevier of Amsterdam (The Netherlands), who produces EMBASE.

158

CCTR contains over 300,000 bibliographic references to controlled trials in health care. Cochrane groups and other organizations contribute their specialized registers; and these registers—together with references to clinical trials identified in MEDLINE and EMBASE—form the CCTR database. Contributors to the Cochrane Collaboration follow quality control standards to ensure that only reports of definite randomized controlled trials or controlled clinical trials are included.

Although many reports of trials are included in MEDLINE, others are not easily identified as randomized controlled trials; and, as such, researchers may overlook them in the search for relevant studies for systematic reviews. CCTR records are identified through a combination of handsearching and database searching that includes all those records indexed as controlled trials in MEDLINE. Studies have shown that a MEDLINE search alone cannot be relied upon to identify all possible reports of controlled trials and suggest that a combination of handsearching and MEDLINE searching is most effective. This dual approach is the current practice of the Cochrane Collaboration, assuring the definitive quality of the CCTR database.

DATABASE OF ABSTRACTS OF REVIEWS OF EFFECTIVENESS (3)

The Database of Abstracts of Reviews of Effectiveness (DARE) is the latest addition to Ovid's growing collection of Evidence-Based Medicine Reviews, which also includes the Cochrane Database of Systematic Reviews and the American College of Physicians (ACP) Journal Club (which consists of the ACP Journal Club from the American College of Physicians–American Society for Internal Medicine [ACP-ASIM] and Evidence-Based Medicine from the BMJ Publishing Group).

DARE is a full text database containing critical assessments of systematic reviews from a variety of medical journals. DARE is produced by the expert reviewers and information staff of the National Health Services' Centre for Reviews and Dissemination (NHS CRD) at the University of York, England, and it consists of structured abstracts of systematic reviews from all over the world. DARE records cover topics such as diagnosis, prevention, rehabilitation, screening, and treatment.

Every word of the document text in DARE is searchable, including references. Searching the DARE Fields describes all of the searchable fields and provides at least one search example for each. Within the Full Text display, hypertext features allow one to display an outline of the document and to move immediately to a selected section, as well as to display complete references cited within the text of a document.

AMERICAN COLLEGE OF PHYSICIANS JOURNAL CLUB (4)

The American College of Physicians (ACP) Journal Club Collection consists of two journals, *ACP Journal Club*, a publication of the American College of Physicians, and *Evidence-Based Medicine*, a joint publication with the British Medical Journal Group.

159

The editors of *ACP Journal Club* screen the top clinical journals on a regular basis and identify studies that are both methodologically sound and clinically relevant. They write an enhanced abstract of the chosen articles and provide a commentary on the value of the article for clinical practice. Using this source, clinicians can quickly understand and apply important changes in medical knowledge to their practice without having to read and synthesize for themselves thousands of journal articles.

Every word of the document text in the ACP Journal Club is searchable, including references, captions, and footnotes. Searching the ACP Journal Club Fields describes all the searchable fields and provides at least one search example for each. The user may also browse the Evidence-Based Medicine and ACP Journal Club publications using the Browse Journals button. Within the Full Text display, hypertext features allow the searcher to display an outline of the document and to move immediately to a selected section, as well as to display complete references cited within the text of a document.

Full text links in the references allow one to explore the evidence in the primary source. Full text references link to other full text documents within the database, as well as to bibliographic databases such as MEDLINE. Bidirectional linking allows linking from MEDLINE to documents in the same collection or to journals available in Ovid Full Text.

ACP Journal Club contains the complete contents of the database dating back to 1991.

REFERENCES

1. *Ovid Cochrane Database Field Guide*. In: Ovid Database Field Guides home page. Available at: http://www.ovid.com/documentation/user/field_guide/ disp_fldguide.cfm?db-cochdb.htm. Accessed June 2002.
2. *Ovid CCTR Field Guide*. In: Ovid Database Field Guides home page. Available at: http://www.ovid.com/documentation/user/field_guide/ disp_fldguide.cfm?db-cctrdb.htm. Accessed June 2002.
3. *Ovid DARE Field Guide*. In: Ovid Database Field Guides home page. Available at: http://www.ovid.com/documentation/user/field_guide/ disp_fldguide.cfm?db-daredb.htm. Accessed June 2002.
4. *Ovid ACP Journal Club Field Guide*. In: Ovid Database Field Guides home page. Available at: http://www.ovid.com/documentation/user/field_guide/ disp_fldguide.cfm?db-acpdb.htm. Accessed June 2002.

APPENDIX B

Other Databases and Resources

The World Wide Web provides access to many free health-related online resources. What follows are brief descriptions of some of the most popular.

NATIONAL LIBRARY OF MEDICINE GATEWAY

Address: http://gateway.nlm.nih.gov/.

The National Library of Medicine (NLM) Gateway is a health information portal that simultaneously searches more than a half-dozen online databases, catalogs, and other resources, including PubMed. One of the key goals of the NLM Gateway is to provide novice or casual searchers with an easy-to-use, one-stop-shopping search site.

The Gateway also can serve as a valuable adjunct to a traditional MEDLINE search because it searches a book and audiovisual catalog (LOCATOR*plus*), meeting abstract collections (e.g., *AIDS Meetings* and *Health Services Research Meetings*), a consumer health site (MEDLINEplus), journal article citations from roughly 1958 through 1965 (OLDMEDLINE), and the Health Services Research Projects database.

Example: Using the NLM Gateway

Locate some OLDMEDLINE articles on the *pulmonary effects of hexametho-nium*. Conduct a broad search with the term *hexamethonium AND (lung OR pul-monary)*. Be sure to use upper case for Boolean operators. The Results Sum-mary will show the number of hits in different categories. To retrieve the OLDMEDLINE citations, click Display Results.

Use the Pick a Collection pull-down menu to select OLDMEDLINE (**A**). Then click the Jump to Collection button (**B**).

The results are displayed below.

For more in-depth or complex searches, use the search interface provided by a specific resource (e.g., PubMed, MEDLINEplus, LOCATORplus).

CLINICALTRIALS.GOV

Address: http://clinicaltrials.gov/.

ClinicalTrials.gov is a repository of information about ongoing clinical trials for "both federally and privately funded trials of experimental treatments for serious or life-threatening diseases or conditions" (1). Multiple search options, each of which is simple and intuitive, are provided.

Example: Using ClinicalTrials.gov

Locate open clinical trials on *vaccine therapy* and *colorectal cancer* while limiting the search to trials in California. Start by selecting Focused Search from the ClinicalTrials.gov home page. Type in the search terms (**A**) and click the Search button (**B**).

Several studies are currently recruiting.

MEDLINEPLUS

Address: http://medlineplus.gov/.

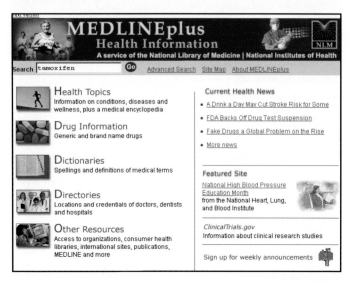

MEDLINEplus provides access to information about diseases and conditions and links to consumer health information from the National Institutes of Health, dictionaries, lists of hospitals and physicians, health information in Spanish and other languages, and clinical trials (2).

The search box, which searches multiple resources simultaneously, is easy to use. Simply type in a term (e.g., *tamoxifen*) and click Go.

MEDLINEplus retrieved information from a wide range of resources. The link to *MEDLINEplus Drug Information: Tamoxifen (Systemic)* is promising.

Select the Tamoxifen link.

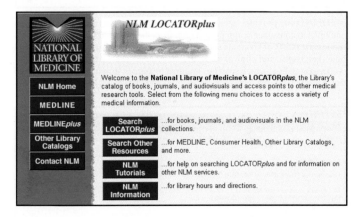

This takes the user to a fairly detailed description of the drug, its side effects, proper use, and other information.

LOCATORPLUS

Address: http://locatorplus.gov/.

LOCATOR*plus* is NLM's online catalog to books, audiovisuals, and journal holdings. Materials are accessible primarily by interlibrary loan (i.e., items can only be requested through the local public or medical library).

Example: Using LOCATORplus

If the user is searching for books on the topic of Celiac Disease, he or she would type *celiac disease* in the search interface, select Title Search (**A**) and Books Only (**B**), and then click Search (**C**).

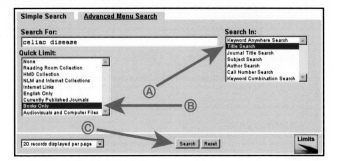

The search retrieved five records.

#	Title	Author	Dates
[1]	Celiac disease : methods and protocols / edited by Michael N. Marsh.		2000
	Library Location: General Collection *Call Number: 2001 E-609*	*Status: Available*	
[2]	Diet and nutrition sourcebook : basic consumer health information about dietary guidelines, recommended daily intake values, vitamins, minerals, fiber, fat, weight control, dietary supplements, and food additives : along with special sections on nutrition		1999
	Title in Multiple Locations		
[3]	Serologic diagnosis of celiac disease / editors, Tadeusz P. Chorzelski ... [et al.].		1990
	Library Location: General Collection *Call Number: WD 175 S486 1990*	*Status: Available*	
[4]	Celiac disease; recipes for parents and patients.	Toronto. Hospital for Sick Children.	1968
	Library Location: General Collection *Call Number: WD 175 T686c 1968*	*Status: Available*	
[5]	Management of celiac disease, by Sidney Valentine Haas and Merrill Patterson Haas.	Haas, Sidney Valentine, 1870-	1951
	Library Location: General Collection *Call Number: WD 175 H112m 1951*	*Status: Available*	

B. OTHER DATABASES AND RESOURCES

PUBMED CENTRAL

Address: http://pubmedcentral.nih.gov/.

PubMed Central is a digital archive of life sciences journal literature managed by the National Center for Biotechnology Information (NCBI) at the U.S. National Library of Medicine (NLM). It is not a journal publisher. Access to PubMed Central (PMC) is free and unrestricted. Learn more about how publishers can participate in PMC.

Available Journals
Click on a Journal Name to see the Table of Contents for the latest available issue. Click in the 'Archive Starts With' column to see a list of all available issues for the journal.

Journal Name	Archive Starts With
Arthritis Research	Vol. 1(1); 1999
BMC Titles [See complete list]	Vol. 1; 2000
bmj.com	Vol. 316(7131); 1998
Breast Cancer Research	Vol. 1(1); 1999
Bulletin of the Medical Library Association	Vol. 88(1); 2000
Cancer Cell International	Vol. 1(1); 2001
CMAJ: Canadian Medical Association Journal	Vol. 163(2); 2000
Critical Care	Vol. 1(1); 1997
Current Controlled Trials in Cardiovascular Medicine	Vol. 1(1); 2000

PubMed Central provides an archive of freely accessible life science journals. Links to PubMed Central journal articles are labeled *Free in PMC* in PubMed.

NATIONAL GUIDELINE CLEARINGHOUSE

Address: http://www.guideline.gov/.

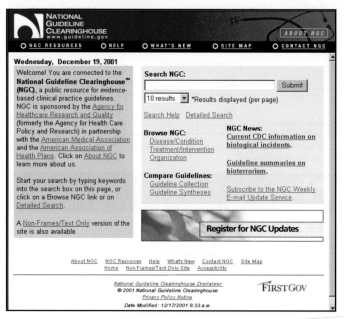

The Agency for Healthcare Research and Quality, in partnership with the American Medical Association and the American Association of Health Plans, created the *National Guideline Clearinghouse* (NGC) as a means of facilitating access to clinical practice guidelines. Each guideline record includes summaries and syntheses of the guideline, including information on the availability of the full text (some records link directly to the full text of the guideline). The Clearinghouse is searchable on the Web at no charge.

Example: Using National Guideline Clearinghouse

If a user is looking for guidelines on the treatment of otitis media with effusion in children, he or she could type *"otitis media" AND effusion AND child**. Click the Submit button.

Several guidelines are relevant.

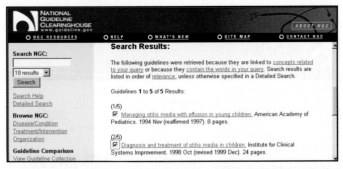

As has been mentioned earlier, some records in NGC provide links to the full text of the guideline.

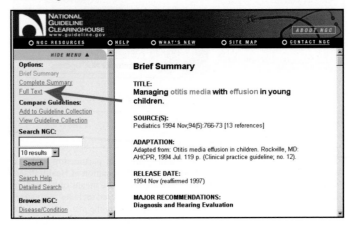

REFERENCES

1. About *ClinicalTrials.gov*. Available at: http://clinicaltrials.gov/info/about. Accessed June 2002.
2. About MEDLINEplus. Available at: http://www.nlm.nih.gov/medlineplus/aboutmedlineplus.html. Accessed June 2002.

Glossary

Abridged Index Medicus (AIM). AIM, which is no longer in print, was a condensed version of *Index Medicus* (see below) that was limited to 120 core clinical journals. The index was designed for small-sized to medium-sized hospitals whose collections, although limited, usually included most of the titles indexed in AIM. AIM now exists as a Subset limit in Ovid MEDLINE as AIM Journals and in PubMed as Core Clinical Journals.

ACP Journal Club. See Appendix A.

AIDSLINE. A database that focuses on the acquired immunodeficiency syndrome/human immunodeficiency virus (AIDS/HIV) literature. The database was recently closed; its journal citations were moved to MEDLINE, its monographic citations to LOCATOR*plus*, and its meeting abstracts to the National Library of Medicine (NLM) Gateway.

Asterisk. Next to a Medical Subject Heading (MeSH) term, the asterisk indicates that the MeSH term is one of the Major Topics of the article. The asterisk is also used as a truncation symbol in PubMed.

AutoAlert. This is one of Ovid's save search options. As a particular database is updated, AutoAlert will run any stored searches against the newly added citations. Citations that match the search profile are then e-mailed to the searcher.

BIOETHICSLINE. BIOETHICSLINE was a database of references dealing with the ethical and legal aspects of health care. The database was recently closed; its journal citations were moved to MEDLINE, its monographic citations to LOCATOR*plus*, and its meeting abstracts to NLM Gateway.

BIOSIS Previews. BIOSIS Previews covers the literature of the biologic and biomedical sciences from 1969 to present. A subscription or fee is required for access.

CANCERLIT. This database covers " . . . cancer therapy, including experimental and clinical cancer therapy; chemical, viral, and other cancer-causing agents; mechanisms of carcinogenesis; biochemistry, immunology, and physiology of cancer; and mutagen and growth factor studies. Some of the information in CANCERLIT is derived from the MEDLINE database. Approximately 200 core journals contribute a large percentage of the records. In addition, other information is drawn from proceedings of meetings, government reports, symposia reports, theses, and selected monographs." *(From the Ovid CANCERLIT Field Guide. Available at: http://ovid.gwdg.de/ovidweb/fldguide/cancer.htm. Accessed June 2002.)*

CAS Registry Numbers. See **Registry Number (RN)**.

Check Tags. Check tags represent general parameters or aspects of the content of a particular article (1). Allegedly, the term *check tags* refers to the days when indexers would manually check-off various tags for each article they indexed.

Check tags include Human, Animal, Male, Female, Case Report, Comparative Study, and others.

Citations. These are short-hand representations of bibliographic works (e.g., books, journal articles). They are sometimes referred to as references or records.

ClinicalTrails.gov. See Appendix B.

Clipboard. A PubMed feature that allows searchers to save selected citations. Duplicate citations are automatically deleted.

Cochrane Database of Systematic Reviews. See Appendix A.

The Cubby. A feature of PubMed that stores search strategies. Searchers can return and rerun stored searches, retrieving only citations added since the last search. The Cubby also provides options for specifying which LinkOut providers are to be displayed in PubMed and for choosing from a list of document delivery services.

Database of Abstracts of Reviews of Effectiveness (DARE). See Appendix A.

EMBASE. EMBASE is a biomedical database similar to MEDLINE. EMBASE is particularly well known for its coverage of the drug research literature. A subscription or fee is required to access the database.

Enzyme Code (EC). The EC is assigned by the Enzyme Commission to represent a particular enzyme. ECs are searchable in MEDLINE.

Explode. This feature of MEDLINE search systems automatically searches a particular medical subject heading and any narrower subject headings. For example, exploding the MeSH Lung Diseases automatically searches Cystic Fibrosis, Pulmonary Edema, and others. Many systems are configured to explode MeSH terms automatically.

Field Tags. These tags represent a particular field within a citation. Although field tags require a modicum of effort to learn, they ultimately can save the searcher some time. For example, running an author search in Ovid by typing *smith j.au* is easier than using the author search icon.

Focus. In Ovid MEDLINE, Focus restricts a medical subject heading search to articles in which that heading is one of the major topics of the article (MeSH terms within the citation will be marked with an asterisk). This is synonymous with PubMed's Restrict Search to Major Topic Headings Only.

Gateway. See **National Library of Medicine (NLM) Gateway**.

Hedge. A hedge is usually a presaved search strategy that a searcher can selectively combine with another search topic. For example, PubMed's Clinical Queries search mode uses a hedge of words and phrases (i.e., randomized controlled trial, drug therapy, therapeutic use, random) to represent the concept of treatment. The searcher then can apply the treatment hedge to a particular disease, such as yellow fever.

Index Medicus. The venerable 120-year-old print index to journals in health and medicine. The contents of *Index Medicus* (1966 to present) are searchable online through MEDLINE. See also **OLDMEDLINE**.

In-Process Citations. More or less synonymous with Ovid's PREMEDLINE, PubMed uses *in-process* to represent citations that are waiting to be indexed with data like medical subject headings, publication types, and so on.

Loansome Doc. This document-ordering service is available through PubMed.

Major Topic. Using this feature restricts a medical subject heading search to articles in which that heading is one of the major topics of the article.

MeSH. See **Medical Subject Headings**.

Medical Subject Headings. Medical Subject Headings, or **MeSH**, consist of more than 19,000 terms that represent an enormous number of concepts ranging from Anterior Cruciate Ligament to Preferred Provider Organizations. The subject headings are arranged hierarchically, with narrower headings falling under broader headings, all of which fall under one or more of 15 supercategories (e.g., Anatomy, Organisms, Diseases, Chemicals and Drugs). For example, under the MeSH term Migraine are the narrower headings Common Migraine and Classic Migraine.

National Library of Medicine (NLM) Gateway. This global search interface and portal provides access to multiple online resources. See Appendix B.

OLDMEDLINE: Available through the NLM Gateway, OLDMEDLINE contains citations from the 1958 through 1965 *Cumulated Index Medicus* (see **Index Medicus**). OLDMEDLINE's citations lack abstracts, and the subject headings (from the 1960 through 1965 MeSH thesaurus) are stored as keywords. For more information, see Appendix B.

Portable Document Format (PDF). PDF is a popular and attractive format for rendering full-text documents. PDF preserves the fonts and formatting of the original document. It is widely preferred to text rendered in hypertext mark-up language (HTML).

Portals. This term represents categorized collections of online resources housed under one roof. Yahoo! is perhaps the best known example of a Web portal; these are sometimes called *horizontal portals*.

PREMEDLINE. In the past, PubMed identified certain citations as *PREMEDLINE*, that is, as citations waiting for indexing before being added to MEDLINE proper. Although PubMed now seems to identify these citations as *in-process*, Ovid still uses the term *PREMEDLINE*. Ovid maintains these citations both as a separate database called PREMEDLINE and as a combination database, *PREMEDLINE + MEDLINE*. PREMEDLINE citations lack MeSH.

173

PsychINFO. This database of psychologic literature covers 1887 to present. A subscription or fee is required for access.

Publication Types. Indexers use this to identify what kind of article is being indexed. More than 40 types exist, including Review, Randomized Controlled Trial, Practice Guideline, and Meta-Analysis.

PubMed Central. The repository, or digital archive, contains free, full-text journal articles. See Appendix B for more information.

PubMed Identification (PMID). PMID is the unique identification number for each citation within PubMed.

Publisher-Supplied Citations. See **Supplied by Publisher**.

Qualifiers. See **Subheadings**.

Records. See **Citations**.

Registry Number (RN). The Chemical Abstracts Service (CAS) Registry Number is a unique number associated with a particular organic or inorganic compound. For example, the CAS registry number for interferon alpha-2b is 99210-65-8. Registry numbers are searchable in MEDLINE.

Registry Number Word (RW). In Ovid MEDLINE, this includes single words from the registry number field, and it can be used to search parts of chemical names (e.g., 15442-64-5 [zinc protoporphyrin]).

Search Set. This term refers to the set of citations resulting from a particular search. For example, an author search on *Morris JD* results in a search set of 43 citations.

Stop Words. Online retrieval systems are required to ignore these common words if they are used as search terms. Typical examples include *of*, *the*, etc.

Subheadings. MEDLINE searchers can use more than 80 subheadings, or qualifiers, to fine-tune a medical subject heading (MeSH) search. Subheadings represent specific aspects of the MeSH term they modify. For example, a searcher can use the subheading Adverse Effects to modify the MeSH term Tamoxifen or can attach Complications to the subject heading Pneumonia, Rickettsial.

    NOTE: PubMed explodes subheadings with *narrower* subheadings. For example, adding the subheading Therapy to the subject heading Crohn Disease will result in Crohn Disease/Therapy, Crohn Disease/Diet Therapy, Crohn Disease/Drug Therapy, Crohn Disease/Nursing, Crohn Disease/Prevention and Control, Crohn Disease/Radiotherapy, Crohn Disease/Rehabilitation, Crohn Disease/Surgery, and Crohn Disease/Transplantation. One can use the Do Not Explode this Term option under Detailed Display to deactivate this feature. In Ovid MEDLINE, the user needs to specify exactly which subheadings to use.

Subsets. Topic, journal, and citation status subsets provide another method for narrowing the scope of the search. For example, the Core Clinical Journals subset limits a search to 120 high-impact clinical journals, most of which are available at small-sized to medium-sized hospital libraries.

Supplied by Publisher. In PubMed, *as supplied by publisher* indicates that citation records were transmitted to the NLM electronically by journal publishers. Most, but not all, of these *eventually* will receive full indexing. Citations that never receive full indexing include (a) out-of-scope articles (e.g., on geology, paleontology) from *selectively* indexed MEDLINE journals and (b) publisher-supplied records from unindexed back issues of the journals (e.g., issues published prior to the acceptance of that journal for inclusion in MEDLINE).

Text Word. In PubMed, Text Word is a broad search that includes the following fields: abstracts, MeSH terms, subheadings, chemical substance names, personal name as subject (e.g., *Pauling L [ps]*), and MEDLINE Secondary Source (databanks and accession numbers of sequences [e.g., GenBank/MP203030]).

Text Word searching in PubMed is similar to "keyword" searching in Ovid, as it includes some of the same fields (e.g., titles, abstracts, and subject headings).

NOTE: The term keyword has a variety of meanings depending on the context in which it is used and the system in which it is searched. In bibliographic database searching, keyword usually refers to a free-text search of multiple fields (e.g., abstract, title, subject headings).

In Ovid MEDLINE, for instance, a keyword search is a simultaneous search of titles, abstracts, CAS Registry and Enzyme Code terms, and Medical Subject Headings (MeSH). In Ovid, the *.mp* field tag is appended to keyword searches (*mp* stands for *multipurpose* because the specific fields it searches vary from database to database).

In addition, some journals require authors to supply keywords or key terms that describe the content of their articles. Several databases (not MEDLINE) will actually make these terms available for searching (e.g., SciSearch, which is a fee-based online version of the Science Citation Index).

Vortals: The online resources contained within vortals, or *vertical portals*, focus on a specific discipline or specialty (as opposed to *horizontal portals* like Yahoo!, which contain many areas of knowledge). Examples include WebMD and Medscape.

REFERENCES

1. National Library of Medicine. *Medical subject headings, annotated alphabetic list, 2001.* Bethesda, MD: The Library, 2001.

SUBJECT INDEX